Set Your Eyes Higher

A 40-Day Reset

TO SLOW YOUR ANXIETY
AND FIX YOUR FOCUS ON GOD

Whitney Lowe

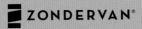

ZONDERVAN

Set Your Eyes Higher

Copyright © 2024 Whitney Lowe

Published in Grand Rapids, Michigan, by Zondervan. Zondervan is a registered trademark of The Zondervan Corporation, L.L.C., a wholly owned subsidiary of HarperCollins Christian Publishing, Inc.

Requests for information should be addressed to customercare@harpercollins.com.

ISBN 978-0-3104-6440-2 (HC)
ISBN 978-0-3104-6443-3 (audiobook)
ISBN 978-0-3104-6441-9 (eBook)

Published in association with The Bindery Agency, www.TheBinderyAgency.com

Art direction: Tiffany Forrester

Interior design: Emily Ghattas

Printed in Vietnam

24 25 26 27 28 SEV 10 9 8 7 6 5 4 3 2 1

Contents

Look
Up.

Introduction

I have always had neck problems. If I sleep at a weird angle on my pillow, or even perform a bicep curl the wrong way, I wake up with a pinched nerve that makes turning my head impossible for weeks. In recent years, my neck issues have only gotten worse. My job as a luxury travel planner, which we'll talk about later, requires me to look at a screen, and my life seems to be increasingly oriented around my phone.

The physical pain we feel when we strain our bodies to constantly look down at our devices has an official term: "tech neck." And that's not the only effect I've been feeling. My posture has fundamentally shifted because my eyes are always looking down. My vision, too, has been compromised by constantly focusing on artificial blue light at close range.

If I want to address the pain, posture, and eyesight strain, I need to set my gaze somewhere else—somewhere up and out. The apostle Paul, whose own vision was profoundly altered by an encounter with the resurrected Christ on the road to Damascus in Acts 9, would agree:

"Since, then, you have been raised with Christ, set your hearts on things above, where Christ is, seated at the right hand of God. Set your minds on things above, not on earthly things. For you died, and your life is now hidden with Christ in God. When Christ, who is your life, appears, then you also will appear with him in glory" (Colossians 3:1–4 NIV).

Paul was writing to the church in Colossae, a city that, at that time, had a significant amount of wealth and economic power living within its walls. The believers there were sincere in their genuine commitment to the gospel. However, likely due to Colossae's proximity to a major trade route, those early Christians were exposed to a diverse range of ideologies and philosophies, and some of these (like Greek asceticism, paganism, and Jewish legalism) became intertwined in the teachings of the Colossian church. This mix of ideas left the Colossians unclear about central Christian truth, and vulnerable to false teachings—particularly those that challenged the deity of Jesus.

That's why Paul wrote to the Colossian church, praising their faith but also advising them to ruthlessly fight back the lies from the culture around them that had started to infiltrate their beliefs. His goal was to reorient the believers at Colossae and remind them to set their eyes back on Christ and His work—to set their eyes higher.

We might not belong to the Colossian church (since, you know, we're a couple thousand years removed from it), but we can gain lots of insight from Paul's letter to this community. There are many parallels between us.

When I look at believers today, I see that so many of us have tons of sincerity and genuine love for God, but I also see cultural influences threatening to skew our focus. I see warped versions of the gospel winning ground in the hearts of Jesus followers. I see believers who claim to be defined by new identities as citizens of a heavenly kingdom tremble with fear of the future. I see them holding contempt for their neighbor and consumed with judgment for others.

Like the Colossians, we're not looking in the right places for guidance. We've been looking down, and all the while, Jesus has been trying to gently grab us by the chin and move our focus back up to Himself.

No, you don't need to keep pursuing perfection on your own. You have already been raised with Christ into holiness.

No, you don't need to live in fear. Jesus has already rescued you from the power of darkness.

No, you don't need to find another source of spiritual enlightenment. The fullness of God dwells in Jesus.

In addition to looking down less, the solution to my neck problems (according to a physical therapist) lies in two practices: 1) daily stretching and 2) retraining my muscles. I think the same exact principles will apply to our spiritual health. We need to shift our gaze back up to the throne of God, and to retrain our mental and spiritual muscles back to healthy functioning. This devotional is a forty-day "boot camp" to doing just that.

I am thankful you are here with me. My goal is that together we will restore our spiritual eyesight so the things of God become clearer, and the lies and distractions fade into the blurry background. Where the latter would leave you discouraged and immobilized, looking to Jesus releases us into joy and radical service. Refocusing our eyes becomes an act of rebellion in a world that is so accustomed to looking downward toward the trivial.

This journey will be split into four key problems I see our generation struggle with most: insecurity, anxiety, burnout, and scarcity. Each of these is the direct result of setting our eyes on the wrong things. We need to be aware of where our gaze has (wrongly) settled, as well as the better thing to turn our eyes unto. As we proceed down this path, you may not get the devotional "warm fuzzies" you're used to—at least not right away. That's okay with me. It's never easy when you lose your focus and have to find it again.

I'd encourage you to commit to reading your Bible every day; that's why each day comes with a suggested passage. Read the Bible for yourself, researching context and letting the Holy Spirit guide you. Along with that, make the effort to open a line of communication between you and Jesus. I'm 100 percent okay if that means a quick prayer like, "God, help!" or, "God, thank You." Prayer can be messy. Lean in. I'd also suggest that you seek at least one person in your life (someone who is actively following Jesus) to talk to whenever you find yourself confused, upset, or in need of some verbal processing. God designed us to follow Him together.

Look up. For there is a good Father who loves you, who made you, who has been trying to get through to you. He is rejoicing over you with singing (Zephaniah 3:17 NIV), if only you could hear it. He is holding you in His strong hands, if only you could feel it. He is sitting on the throne, victorious over all the things coming for your heart, if only you could see it. The first step is to look up, to set your eyes higher.

PART 1

Identity + Insecurity

Our individualistic, modern American culture says if we want to know who we are, we just need to look within. The problem is: I've tried that. And looking at myself isn't helping. I either find myself consumed with my imperfections or altogether avoiding my flaws.

On the other hand, I have always found it confusing when Christians say, "My identity is in Christ." What, exactly, does that entail? I want us to dig into this idea together: If Jesus is supposed to be the basis for how we define ourselves, what does it really mean for Jesus to be the Source and Sustainer of who you are?

Over the next ten days, we're going to gain a deeper under-standing of a few ways we're erroneously seeking to form our identity, and instead, how we can derive our value and worth in our relationship with God. Together, let's reset our vision on His unshifting nature and find stability in His faithfulness.

Set your eyes on His image, and come into alignment with who He created you to be.

> For in him all things were created: things in heaven and on earth, visible and invisible, whether thrones or powers or rulers or authorities; all things have been created through him and for him. He is before all things, and in him all things hold together.
>
> **Colossians 1:16–17** NIV

Set
your
eyes
on
His
image.

1

Approval Over Everything

In 2019, God led me to start @scribbledevos, an Instagram account dedicated to theologically robust devotionals and graphics to accompany them. Young women I knew kept telling me they were stressed, sad, scared, and lonely and that they had no time to read their Bibles or pray. They also seemed to spend hours on their phones scrolling social media. From day one, the goal of @scribbledevos was to disrupt that scroll with truth—to give them a little nudge toward setting their eyes higher.

When I told them about my Instagram account, these young women all followed me, and their lives were changed forever.

Ha, just kidding! I was too scared to share my writing and too afraid for people to have a window into my heart. I kept this side project a total secret for months. What I didn't expect is that the idea would catch on. It turns out people actually *liked* seeing devotionals on their feed. They liked the graphics I was scrambling to put together on the fly every day. All of a sudden, I had "a following."

Allow me to share a small secret: I am an approval *junkie*. I have spent my whole life trying to ensure that people will like me. If I sense people getting close to discovering my flaws, I put up a wall; better to be admired from a distance than truly known up close. And so, as I followed this nudge from God to create @scribbledevos, I also set myself on a crash course with all of my insecurities and fears.

I was agonizing over typos in my caption, because I was afraid they would made me look dumb. I'd find myself frustrated to the point of tears when I was misunderstood by an angry commenter. I tracked how many followers I lost because losing followers felt like the ultimate failure.

In the social media landscape, we are led to believe that if we don't have followers, we must be doing something wrong. We buy into the lie that our identity is appraised based on how much approval we can win. We start to believe that our inherent value comes from others' perceptions of us.

As God has used @scribbledevos to (I hope!) bless other people on the internet, He's used it to demolish my obsession with others' approval and my desperate desire to feel like I was worth following.

I hope this lesson saves you from the many tears I cried as I learned it the hard way: I am only worth following to the extent that I point you (yes, *you*!) to Jesus, the singular Source of life, joy, and peace. My identity is not caught up in others' approval but in His.

And guess what? Following Jesus isn't always glamorous and Instagrammable. Following Jesus fundamentally challenges our desire to be comfortable and our desire to be accepted:

"Then he called the crowd to him along with his disciples and said: 'Whoever wants to be my disciple must deny themselves and take up their cross and follow me'" (Mark 8:34 NIV).

Here, Jesus was teaching His disciples—His followers—about the suffering and rejection He would endure before His brutal execution and miraculous resurrection three days later. Peter seemed to understand what Jesus was saying, and he wanted nothing of it. Mark tells us that Peter actually rebuked Jesus for saying this (the audacity!). And here, friends, is where we get those famous, fear-invoking words from the mouth of our gentle Savior: "'Get behind me, Satan!' he said. 'You do not have in mind the concerns of God, but merely human concerns'" (Mark 8:33 NIV).

Ouch. Following Jesus, it turns out, often leads us down the inherently unpopular path of rejection and suffering. When we fight that reality, we end up positioning ourselves in opposition to Jesus, just like Peter did here. If we need followers and approval to feel good about who we are, we simply preclude the possibility of our identities ever being found in Jesus Christ.

Take your eyes off others' approval and your follower count—real or metaphorical. Make peace with the fact that Jesus didn't call you to win others' opinions, and realize that disapproval won't kill you. Set your eyes, instead, on the cross Jesus calls you to carry. I bet you'll be shocked by how many people join you.

Dear God,

I confess that sometimes I want the approval of others more than I want Yours. I sometimes want to gain followers more than I want to follow You. Help me find my identity in You, not in the acceptance of people. Help me, Lord.

Amen.

2

Who Are You Following?

Today I'm going to introduce you to one of the most significant influences on my faith since I was twelve years old: Lisa.

When I met Lisa, she was twenty-three—a time when many of us are too preoccupied figuring out our own lives to give back to others. But she gave up time, money, and *significant* emotional energy so that a few teenage girls might come to love Jesus more. For six years, beginning in the seventh grade, she met with me and my two best friends twice a week. A few years into our study together, one of our weekly meetings was a six a.m. Bible study in a bagel shop across the street from our high school. We would sit at a table in the corner and talk about our lives, read a chapter of the Bible aloud, discuss it, and pray for each other.

I dreaded it.

No, not the early wakeup call. That part was fine. I also loved catching up with my friends, and I loved talking about the Bible. The part that made my fifteen-year-old skin crawl was

My
identity
is not
caught up
in others'
approval.

when we would pray aloud in an otherwise silent Einsteins Bros. Bagels. The only other patrons were keeping quietly to themselves. As the morning went on, more and more of our classmates filled the shop, and I would catch their side-eye glances while they eavesdropped.

I should also add that Lisa is *loud*. If you met her, you'd know her famous laugh—the kind that makes strangers on the opposite side of the room laugh too. She's not the type to overthink others' perceptions of her, and she certainly does not waste a thought on earning others' approval. I, on the other hand, was deeply self-conscious and, at times, even ashamed. *Couldn't we just pray in private? Or at least in a whisper?* I was concerned with the approval of others. She didn't define herself based on what others thought of her, but by following Christ and helping others do the same.

We could all be more like Lisa. I used to find my identity in the opinions of other people, but I now know that being saved by Jesus is the core of my identity, and I want others to know it too. I've learned to resist the urge to prove that I am "cool" or perfect, and I focus on using my gifts to serve and love other people, even if it makes me a little (or a lot) nervous.

Following Jesus requires an identity shift. Our identities are defined by following Him.

Look at Jesus' own disciples:

"As Jesus was walking beside the Sea of Galilee, he saw two brothers, Simon called Peter and his brother Andrew. They were casting a net into the lake, for they were fishermen. 'Come, follow me,' Jesus said, 'and I will send you out to fish for people.' At once they left their nets and followed him" (Matthew 4:18–20 NIV).

Fishing was the family trade for Peter and Andrew, and in the days of Jesus, it would have been central to their identity. Leaving their family business would have been scandalous, even reckless in the eyes of their community. But Jesus calls them to leave it all behind—and they do. (Imagine the side-eye glances *they* would have received!) But this kind of boldness isn't reserved just for Jesus' early disciples; Jesus calls *all* of us to this kind of boldness, the kind that could not care less who hears you praying loudly in a bagel shop.

Your identity has never been tied to how many followers you can win (online or IRL in an Einstein's Bros.). It's not about looking impressive and gaining the approval of others around you. Your identity has everything to do with whom you choose to follow.

Like Lisa and those very first disciples, can we decentralize ourselves and elevate Jesus as the only One worth following? Jesus is calling us to leave behind the nets of approval-seeking that are holding us back and instead to fully embrace the reality that who we are is hidden in who He is (Colossians 3:3–4 NIV). Our identity is most fully realized when we are making Jesus known.

What's holding you back from embracing that call?

Dear Lord,
I want to follow You with all that I am, and I want to bring others with me. Free me from my need to gain others' approval, and from the lie that I need to build my own following. I want to build Your following, Jesus, and to build up Your kingdom. You alone are worthy.
Amen.

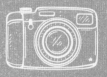

GOD ISN'T CALLING YOU
TO LIVE A FILTERED LIFE.

Filtering Ourselves

My skin care routine *must be working!* I remember thinking to myself. *My face looks brighter, and my cheekbones look more defined.*

I soon realized (though not soon enough to save my pride) that I had accidentally turned on one of those filters that plumps your lips and contours your skin. And I surprised myself with how disappointed I was to see what my face *actually* looked like, sans filter. Forming an accurate, healthy self-image in the age of smartphones and social media is tough work. In many ways, our sense of identity has been reduced to how we look on a phone screen.

With infinite ways to Photoshop and filter and perfect our images, we're living our *entire lives* through a curated lens. I am so accustomed to filtering my life experiences through highlight reels that I find myself less interested in going places that aren't Instagrammable or, heaven *forbid*, allowing my skin to show my years and the hard-won lines of motherhood.

Social media offers us a flimsy idea of identity. It serves us the praise we covet ("You're beautiful!" or "I wish I were you!"), and it leaves us hungry for more. When our posts don't get enough likes, our minds go into overdrive over *why*. When someone writes a gushing comment, we get a weird little high. Here is my question: What if the best "you" that you could present—the "flawless" version— still doesn't get the attention and affirmation you crave? If people online don't even like the idealized version of you, then what?

Deriving our value from likes and clicks and comments is a fruitless way to form a sense of self. No wonder we're so exhausted! We have bought into the lie that if we're not "perfect" or "likable" by the ever-changing standards of the world, then we are not valuable. But Jesus is the only One who has ever been perfect—and let's remember, He was described to be not particularly physically striking (Isaiah 53:2 NIV). So why do we spend so much time curating an online persona and image? Why is it so easy to slip into patterns of trying to convince others that we're without flaw or error? Why are we wasting so much time, frankly, telling a lie?

If we want to break ourselves from these vicious patterns of approval-seeking, we need to get clear on where our value comes from. In the book of Genesis, we read, "God created mankind in his own image" (1:27 NIV). Right here in the very first book of the Bible, we learn our identity—we are image bearers of a holy, wondrous God. Yes, we fall and we fail, but that inherent goodness is in our DNA, however obscured it may be at times.

Your worth is set for all eternity. Your identity is directly linked to God's own image. If you're fixating on getting validation while pretending to be someone you're not, you're missing it. God isn't calling you to live a filtered life; He is calling you to live an authentic one that bears witness to Him. If your heart is so consumed with trying to appear perfect and fit in, you're pursuing an image that God didn't create you for. God made you in His image, yet you're striving to mold yourself into the image of something lesser.

He will do more transformative work in your life than any filter ever could, and all you have to do is show up exactly as you are. A good, kind Creator knit you together with His goodness, and He wants to bring that work to completion (Philippians 1:6 NIV). Being a Christian means being messy; it's actually a prerequisite to walking this path. All God asks of you is to bring your mess to Him.

This quest for perfection—the editing, the filtering, the curating, and the (I hate to say it) lying—is an anxiety-ridden distraction from your true identity made in the image of God. You have a God who desires a wholly unfiltered relationship with you, promising to love you no matter what you say or do. And He will never, ever ask you to clean yourself up before you come to Him.

Lord,
I have believed the lie that I can make myself perfect. I have spent time and energy and resources trying to project a false reality, all because I am desperate to feel worthy. I concede that my best attempt at perfect isn't cutting it. Help me to shift my gaze off my perfection and remember the value You have already given me.
Amen.

4

Flawed Heroes

One of my favorite passages in the Bible is Hebrews 11, sometimes referred to as the "Hall of Faith." It celebrates the figures in the Old Testament who trusted God, and it's a beautiful testament to what God can do through His people. That's not why I like it though. I like it because everyone listed in this chapter is deeply flawed. If you are prone to perfectionism like me, you might find this freeing . . . or incredibly frustrating.

Abraham and Sarah are lauded for following God without knowing where they were going, and for trusting Him for their promised child in their old age. This is the same Abraham who twice claimed Sarah as his sister instead of his wife to preserve his own life (a key indicator that he did not, in fact, trust God with this future). And Sarah? She laughed in disbelief when she found out she would become pregnant.

Noah is in the Hall of Faith for obediently building an ark before seeing a drop of rain. The same Noah later got so drunk that he was disgraced.

Then there is Moses, one of the most central figures in Israel's history, celebrated for looking ahead to his reward instead of living in comfort as a prince of Egypt. And yet, he was not allowed to enter the promised land because he shortsightedly disobeyed God's direct words.

The Hall of Faith is, then, a picture of how God chooses to redeem broken people and messy stories. These individuals were not perfect by any stretch of the imagination, but Hebrews 11 says their faith was credited as righteousness. Through faith in God, the people we would call villains become heroes. That's what happens when you put your identity in Christ. And I assure you that same redemption is still at work in *you* today.

Paul (a mass murderer, I might add) explained it this way: "But he said to me, 'My grace is sufficient for you, for my power is made perfect in weakness.' Therefore I will boast all the more gladly about my weaknesses, so that Christ's power may rest on me. . . . For when I am weak, then I am strong" (2 Corinthians 12:9–10 NIV). Scholars still debate what Paul's weakness was, but the point is this: God chose him—a murdering, "weak" man—to bring the gospel to the Gentiles.

So how did these flawed individuals end up as the heroes of the faith?

Jesus, who knew no sin, was made to be sin on our behalf. Jesus, who is seated in heaven at the right hand of God, came to earth to experience our every ailment and temptation. God sees us as His children, regardless of how problematic our past or how difficult our current struggles.

This is what frees us: Jesus has made us perfect before God, so we can stop trying to achieve it. In fact, if we want to experience

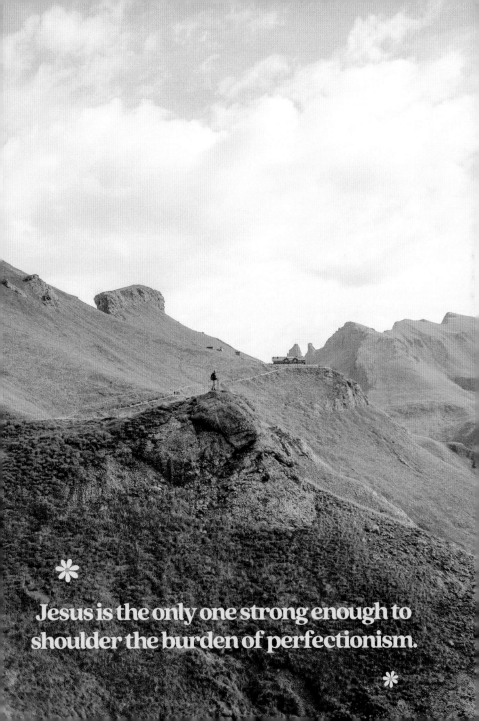

Jesus is the only one strong enough to shoulder the burden of perfectionism.

the kind of radical power that we see in the Hall of Faith, we must stop trying to hide our flaws and instead give them to God.

Jesus is the only one strong enough to shoulder the burden of perfectionism. Embrace that reality, and find peace. Lay down that burden, because it's crushing you. Give yourself a chance to witness how powerfully God moves in our gaps.

If we could just zoom out from our own faces, our own résumés, our own personality flaws and the immense effort we're using to force them into perfection, *then* maybe we would see that Jesus is right there, just above our eyeline. We're trying to mold the messy, misshapen clay of our lives into a Renaissance sculpture by sheer willpower and manipulation, while the God of the universe is standing right there, proving from the very beginning that He makes beautiful things out of *dust* (Genesis 2:7). Unfortunately, for perfectionists like myself, we must first recognize that we are, at our core, that same dust. But, oh, what God can do when we give up the pursuit of perfection we will never achieve and let Him work our mess into a masterpiece. There is nothing God can't do with surrendered dust.

Lord,
Thank You for being perfect so I can stop trying to be. Thank You for freeing me from the burden of flawlessness. Thank You for covering me with Your perfection so that I can be near to You. Help me keep my eyes on all the ways You have redeemed my imperfection instead of on all the ways I don't measure up. Help me walk in that freedom.
Amen.

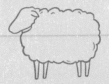

GOD IS A GOOD SHEPHERD.

5

The Peace
of a Sheep

When I was in seventh grade, I gave my best attempt at an "edgy phase." We had just moved back to Colorado from a short stint in Florida, and this would be my first year of middle school after a year of homeschool and a cross-country move. I felt pressure to show that I was still "normal," and I probably overcorrected. And I really committed to this phase—skater shoes, studded belts, heavy eyeliner. I downloaded the most popular hardcore rock songs I knew at that time: a short list, but I did my best. And I spent one hundred dollars (roughly two grand in seventh grade dollars) on a skateboard.

But underneath, I was the same old me—a sweet Christian girl, who went to camp for a month every summer and learned about the Bible. I was just trying out a new identity, telling my family, "This is who I am now!" They knew the truth, of course. I was still obsessed with glitter and devouring The Princess Diaries books in my spare time. I must have looked ridiculous to my parents.

I think our attempts to define ourselves apart from God must look similar. We go around trying on new identities, and meanwhile, the One who knows us better than anyone looks lovingly upon us, waiting for us to come back to our senses.

We may think we want to be the master of our own identities. All of my favorite princess movies from when I was a little girl told the heroine to "follow your heart," and that message rooted itself deep into me! The problem with this mantra is that it assumes that 1) the desires of our hearts are easily understandable, and 2) they can't steer us wrong.

The prophet Jeremiah has some thoughts on this dilemma: "The heart is deceitful above all things, and desperately sick; who can understand it? 'I the Lord search the heart and test the mind'" (Jeremiah 17:9–10 esv).

Sure, you can follow your heart, but what if your heart is lying? What if your heart is sick? What if who you think you are isn't rooted in the identity God designed for you? Since we cannot be sure that our hearts are moving toward God, we should be cautious to follow them. In fact, we should be the *most* careful following what "feels right": some of the most destructive things that exist feel really, really good . . . until they don't.

Any attempt to design our own identity apart from God inevitably lands us in a place of inauthenticity, not truth and freedom. Instead of trying to look at our deceptive, sick hearts to lead us forward, we must look to God to find peace in our identity.

We have to submit ourselves to the truth that God is God—and we are not. We have to surrender to the frustrating but ultimately freeing reality that He knows everything, and we only know a tiny fraction. We have to make peace with the reality that He is the Shepherd and we are sheep. If we can get our heads around these principles, we might stand a chance of truly discerning what God made us to be.

So, I am a sheep. As a Christian, that's my identity. Sometimes I want to shed this identity—I want to be a glittery princess on a noble quest to find herself. That is, until I realize that no quest is more rewarding than the simplicity of following my Shepherd wherever He would lead.

God is a good Shepherd who leads His flock into peace and rest. When I wander, He leaves the entire flock to come find me. Walking with Him, I lack nothing. I know true love in this relationship, trusting that He will protect me and provide His loving goodness forever more.

The older I get, the more sure I am that this Shepherd can truly be trusted. He leads me to better places than I lead myself. In the quest to understand who we are, we are far better off looking to the Creator of our hearts than to our hearts themselves. Looking inward may seem like the solution, but to really understand ourselves, looking up at the staff of the Good Shepherd who is leading you to rest is the only way to go.

God,

I confess my habit of telling You, my Creator,
who I am. But of course You already know
the real me better than anyone. Help me to be
content with being Your sheep, and remind me
that You are such a trustworthy Shepherd.

Amen.

6

Becoming More You

Jesus didn't change Saul's name to Paul. Though the Bible provides powerful examples of God meaningfully renaming people, Paul isn't one of them. Saul was just Paul's Hebrew name, and Paul was his Greek name. Saul probably started to go by Paul because after his dramatic conversion, his ministry largely focused on Gentiles, who spoke Greek.

While Paul certainly went through some significant transformation in his life, Jesus already knew who He had created Paul to be. When the scales fell from his eyes and his sight was restored in Acts 9:18, Paul's true, God-given identity was restored to him too. He was immediately baptized, and he devoted the remainder of his life to making Jesus' name known, no matter what adversity he faced.

Paul didn't need to *change* his name or identity; he needed to turn from sin and live in the God-given identity he had all along. In his conversion, Paul became even *more* himself and *more* aligned with his purpose—to love God and love others. His identity wasn't changed when he met Jesus; it was simply revealed.

After his conversion, Paul threw himself into living out the identity given to him directly by Jesus to be His "chosen instrument to proclaim [His] name" (Acts 9:15 NIV). He knew that Jesus was the most important thing about him. He counted his qualifications as "garbage, that [he] may gain Christ and be found in him" (Philippians 3:8–9 NIV). In fact, some scholars even think that he chose to go by "Paul" because in Greek it means "little." Paul wanted his own identity to be small in comparison to Christ at work in and through him.

Paul considered his identity to be all about who he was following—Jesus, his Lord and Savior. Everything else was secondary, and he trusted God to work out the rest.

We love to look inward (through personality tests and mindfulness practices) or outward (to our social groups or personal relationships) to receive a sense of identity, but both are woefully inadequate on their own and will perpetuate our insecurity because they can't really describe who we are. To really know ourselves, we first must look up to the One who made us.

> You have searched me, LORD, and you know me.
> You know when I sit and when I rise;
> you perceive my thoughts from afar.
> You discern my going out and my lying down;
> you are familiar with all my ways. . . .
> For you created my inmost being;
> you knit me together in my mother's womb.
>
> **Psalm 139:1–3; 13** NIV

I can't tell you all of who you are. But I know some of the basics: You, friend, were made in the image of God.

You were blessed to be a blessing. The good He has knit into you is there to bring about good for others.

You are gifted. God has anointed you with skills and abilities that, when directed by His Spirit, can change lives and impact history.

You are unique. The specific makeup of your brain, the circumstances you come from, where you find yourself now—like Paul—God has both orchestrated and redeemed your particular life for a particular purpose that no one else can fulfill in the same way.

God doesn't need you to know everything about who you are for Him to use you. God doesn't ask us to categorize ourselves according to the hundreds of boxes our society has to offer. God doesn't put the heavy burden of self-definition upon us.

It's okay (and even beneficial!) to contemplate your identity. What I want you remember today is that you are free from the pressure of having to figure it out yourself. God knows all the beauty within you and all the struggles you're wrestling with. Continue to explore your identity and even ask questions. But release the need to tie a pretty bow on your identity, calling it complete.

God implants identity within us from the moment we are created, and then, with each turn in the road, He illuminates just a little bit more of it—a beautiful journey in progress. Embrace the freedom of this divine process.

Lord,
You only make masterpieces, and You are
making me still. My eyes have been locked in
on trying to understand myself and where
I fit in Your kingdom, but You have already
done that work for me. Thank You for the
beauty of the identity You have already given
me; give me the faith to stay close to You
while You work out Your purposes for it.
Amen.

Eyes Down

"**Moooooooooo**," my classmate bellowed, looking me directly in the eye. "Get off the table, cow!"

I was twenty years old, sitting on a coffee table while I was working on a group project. I am sure this fellow student would claim he was only kidding with me, but I can still hear his taunt ringing in my ears.

I was a religious studies major spending a semester abroad in Istanbul, Turkey. We traveled the route of Paul's missionary journeys, reading the letters to the churches mentioned in Revelation as we stood in their very ruins and learning about the ancient church councils right where they had convened. We closed the semester with a month in Israel and Palestine. I was experiencing these beautiful cultures through their local foods, and yes, I had gained a little weight.

The cow remark was rough, but the groundwork for my eating disorder was laid a long time before that. My whole life I had been told I was gifted, but I couldn't have felt less so in the presence of my high-achieving peers. I felt so overlooked, so uninteresting. I was

41

IT'S HARD TO GROW
WHEN YOU'RE OBSESSED
WITH BEING SMALL.

desperate to feel worthwhile, and I eventually found that I could manufacture admiration from people through my appearance.

Instead of taking full advantage of the incredible growth my education and travels had afforded me, I spent much of my college experience looking straight down: at my stomach, my thighs, my calorie-counting app, and my scale. I didn't want to grow; I wanted to shrink. I didn't want dimension; I wanted to be flat. This desire to shrink adversely affected my mind as well as my body. It's hard to grow when you are obsessed with being small.

And isn't this exactly what our society promotes? We spend our days looking at 2D images of perfect people on tiny phone screens. The fashion industry preaches body positivity and inclusivity while manufacturing and promoting products mostly for thin bodies. It's harder than ever to feel comfortable in our skin, and to top it off, we have to conceal our struggles because our culture likes to pretend that it honors all bodies equally.

Perhaps, like me, you've realized that you were not designed to live with your eyes set on the scale or the tags on your clothes. These cultural markers of beauty that we spend so much time obsessing over? They don't determine our worth or our character. Hear me now that I've waded through this struggle myself: this anxiety about your appearance is a waste of your energy.

Jesus knew that too: "Therefore I tell you, do not worry about your life, what you will eat or drink; or about your body, what you will wear. Is not life more than food, and the body more than clothes? Look at the birds of the air; they do not sow or reap or store away in barns, and yet your heavenly Father feeds them. Are you not much more valuable than they? Can any one of you by worrying add a single hour to your life? . . . So do not worry, saying, 'What shall we eat?' or 'What shall we drink?' or 'What shall we wear?'" (Matthew 6:25–27, 31 NIV).

I remember reading this passage through the lens of my eating disorder during my college years. I knew Jesus was speaking to hungry people, not exactly those struggling with bulimia the way I was. But I found so much truth—and hope—in Jesus' words here: you can't add a single hour to your life by agonizing over your appearance.

The lie that you can and should obtain meticulous control over your body is a futile, painful distraction from the work God has set in advance for you to do. There is so much more to living than fitting into a generic, unattainable version of beauty.

What you bring to the world will not be improved by obsessing over the scale.

Your identity is already infused with the beauty of God's image; your efforts to meet cultural beauty standards will only exhaust you.

Jesus tells the crowd to look at the birds flying over their heads. He directs their gaze to God's good and beautiful design, to His generous provision. "Look up," He said. So, let's.

Lord,
Give us the faith to gaze on these bodies You
have given us with gratitude. Help us surrender
our insecurity, knowing that You created us
for more than diet plans and fitness regimens.
Help us identify the lies of our culture and call
them what they are. Lord, help us look up.
Amen.

8

Rare Beauty

I was sitting in a kid-sized plastic chair, sweating in a seventh-floor walkup awash in the June heat of Istanbul, surrounded by small children from Syria, Eritrea, and Sudan. One of them, whose bright eyes I will never forget, was only eighteen months old and had a severe case of cerebral palsy. All of them were refugees. All of them were hungry. There was a lot of need in this room, and a lot of pain.

I was back in Turkey three years after my study abroad experience to serve for a summer with a ministry that, at this point in time, was responding to the refugee crisis caused by the Syrian civil war. Every Monday and Wednesday we hosted a kids' club where moms would bring their children for an activity and a good meal.

Sitting in that tiny chair, I watched these kids devour whatever food we could serve them, which that day was cheese crackers. I watched moms—many of them breastfeeding—give up their portion of food for their hungry kids. I was hungry too, for a different reason: I was secretly still battling my eating disorder.

The irony (and the Holy Spirit) hit me like a brick in that

moment. I was choosing—hoping—to waste away, while these mothers and children were doing anything in their power to survive. I was constantly faint from the heat during the meal service and cleanup. I was not able to serve well because, in my mind, starving myself for thinness was more ideal than nourishing myself for wellness.

A painfully bright lightbulb went on, blinding me just long enough to reset my vision.

My eating disorder began in Istanbul, and my healing did too. God lovingly wrenched my gaze away from myself and shifted my perspective.

In Ephesians 2, Paul basically told us that we have been created as God's masterpieces. As a woman who has struggled with eating disorders, this truth feels so healing, albeit unbelievable at times. But Paul didn't stop there. He said, "For we are God's handiwork, *created in Christ Jesus to do good works*, which God prepared in advance for us to do" (v. 10 NIV, emphasis added).

You are a masterpiece, but you are not here just to look pretty. You are a masterpiece with great purpose. You are a masterpiece meant to do good for other masterpieces. You are a masterpiece, but you will not inhabit the fullness of what that means until you are doing the good works God designed for you.

Many of us have internalized the belief that being beautiful (whatever that means according to the ever-evolving standards of the day) is the most important thing we can be, at any cost and no matter the means. People spend thousands of dollars on a litany of products and procedures to eliminate any perceived flaw. People hyperfixate on perfecting tiny muscle groups and whitening

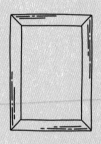

YOU ARE A MASTERPIECE.

already-white teeth one more shade. People like me start to believe the only way to achieve beauty is to starve themselves.

But the kind of beauty God has woven into you? That beauty is meant to bless others. The masterpiece God has made you is at its fullest, brightest, and most beautiful when it's loving and serving.

God's kind of beauty is meant to be understood in conjunction with your mind and your heart. God's kind of beauty is holistic in its essence. To try and attain physical beauty while neglecting your spiritual condition is entirely futile. You are His masterpiece; in every segment of your DNA there is beauty and purpose, inextricably linked.

Diet plans and wrinkle prevention aren't necessarily bad or sinful. But they can become a threat to your physical and spiritual well-being when you become *obsessed* with them. When you find yourself nitpicking your body in self-criticism, begin to shift your gaze from your own insecurity and onto the real needs of the people around you. Then, take delight in God's provision, and nourish yourself—yes, literally! As you are nourished both physically in your body and spiritually in your identity in Christ, over time you will find renewed energy and purpose to nourish others.

God,
Reframe my idea of beauty. Instill into
the deepest part of my heart that I am Your
masterpiece, and in that, I am inherently
beautiful and inherently purposeful. Show
me how I can live into this reality today. I want
Your vision for Your creation and not my own.
Amen.

Blind Spots

"God made you beautiful!" I explained to
a circle of middle school girls—just the words I needed to hear
when I was twelve. "And Jesus died for you!" They looked at me
wide-eyed. I could tell my best efforts to connect with them weren't
landing the way I'd hoped. Oh well, moving on. "Does anyone
have prayer requests?"

One girl—let's call her Maya—raised her hand. "My dad has
cancer, but my mom says we can't afford the treatment. So pray my
dad gets better."

The room went quiet. I knew I should pray and share an
encouraging Bible verse about God's healing power or something.
But the heaviness of this prayer request knocked all the usual
Christian responses right out of me.

We were in a multi-purpose room at a low-income housing
complex in Santa Barbara, California, near my college. My friend
and I—church girls through and through—volunteered to host a
Bible study for the girls living there. We were sure we could make

an impact teaching them about "standard" middle school girl topics. Our blind spots were *massive.*

We were naive. At nineteen years old, we didn't understand how layers of privilege and limited life perspective had formed our faith along narrow lines (upper-middle-class, non-denominational white evangelicalism). Because we didn't acknowledge our own identity and context, we didn't understand why this diverse, low-income community might not find our messaging as relevant. We assumed the needs of this community would be the same as the youth groups we had come from.

Not too long after, Maya tragically lost her dad. She endured more loss and financial anxiety than we had at twice her age. Through all of it, we were made acutely aware of how ill-equipped we truly were to help her.

For one thing, it's nearly impossible to connect with others when you have an inaccurate sense of your own identity and context. As Paul said, "If anyone thinks they are something when they are not, they deceive themselves" (Galatians 6:3 NIV). Paul was instructing the Galatians on living in community, and the principle rings true: if you don't have an accurate, honest grip on who you are, you will not be able to relate honestly to God and others.

First John 4:10–11 explains it well: "This is love: not that we loved God, but that he loved us and sent his Son as an atoning sacrifice for our sins. Dear friends, since God so loved us, we also ought to love one another" (NIV). Notice the progression in this verse: First, we look to God for an honest view of His love for us, because that is what defines us.

Then, since God so loved us, we are compelled, in an honest

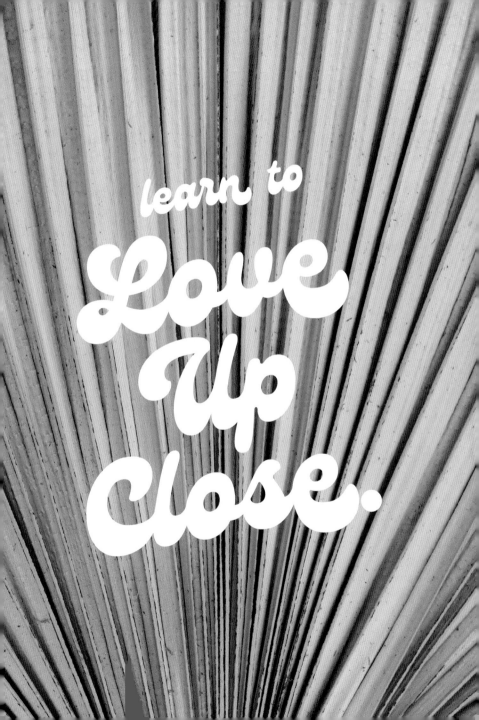

expression of our redeemed spiritual DNA, to love others. Did you catch that? Loving others well is at the core of your identity, because it is at the core of the identity of the God you serve. God is love. Genuine love and service to others starts with an honest, accurate understanding of ourselves.

Once I registered how little I understood about the reality these girls were living in, it enabled me to look for ways to genuinely serve them from a place of humility. Maya needed a place to vent and a space to be a middle school kid, not a lecture on self-esteem. For one hour a week, I could offer her at least that.

Likewise, Jesus' ministry was all about knowing people—where they came from, what made them unique, what ailed them. His love was specific to every person He met. Jesus spent much of His time just getting to know people, dining with anyone who would have Him in their homes. He honored their individual identities and contexts.

"By this everyone will know that you are my disciples, if you love one another," Jesus said in John 13:35 (NIV). In Jesus' own words, love is who you are. It is in receiving and extending His love that we will finally experience the identity alignment we're looking for.

Let yourself get caught up in the love of God, and let it overflow to others in ways that reach them where they are. Learn to love up close, and embrace a fuller identity living out your calling in Christ.

Lord,
I want to love and serve people the way
You did, with an eye on their God-given
dignity and God-rendered uniqueness. I
want to meet real needs. Shed light on my
blind spots so I can see myself accurately
and serve others the way You would.
Amen.

Living Out Love

This year I wasn't planning to give up anything for Lent. In the past, I've given up social media, sugar, coffee, or TV, and it has always helped me direct my focus to Jesus in the weeks leading up to Easter. But as a mom of two, I'm on a never-ending crash course in self-control, so this year I was just fine sitting Lent out.

Cut to a few weeks later. I was standing in line at the grocery store, having successfully avoided all human interaction. I was antsy to get through the self-checkout line with two fussy babies. I just wanted to get home.

In that moment, I heard the Holy Spirit say, "Give up self-checkout for Lent." *Um, pardon?* If it wasn't so completely unlike anything I would ever say, I would have written off this sentence as a rambling of my chronically sleep-deprived subconscious.

So I got in line at one of the human-operated registers. While I unloaded my groceries and braced myself for toddler whining, a few things became clear:

There were hundreds of people in this store I would prefer to ignore.

The idea of my kids melting down in public made me feel vulnerable, and I didn't want others to judge my parenting skills.

I valued efficiency and convenience more than the opportunity to show God's love to other people.

By the time I got to the front of the line, I begrudgingly agreed with God that I would make an effort to be social with my cashier. Today, it was Sally—a middle-aged woman who looked annoyed that I would ask her about her day.

But I pressed anyway. "Do you have anything fun going on this weekend?"

"No."

"Wow, is it always this busy on Thursdays?"

"I don't know. I guess."

I decided to give her a break. I shifted my focus to my toddler, who was begging for candy thanks to the evil geniuses who stock chocolate next to the register.

In that pause, Sally said, "My husband and I had a huge fight this morning. I would much rather be here, actually." She started the sentence trying to make a joke, but it was still too raw. I could see her tears welling up. Something had broken open.

I didn't pry about the nature of the fight. But I did look her in the eye and say, "I am so sorry. I know how that feels. I will be praying that things are better later." I don't know if I helped her, but I did offer connection. Now, when I see Sally at the grocery store, we pick up where we left off.

When we stop looking at only our needs, we can see that opportunities to serve others are right in front of our faces, just inches away, really. If Christ has truly transformed us, that change will overflow into how we engage with others, even in these seemingly insignificant moments.

If you want to learn more about how this transformation can impact your relationship with others, read Colossians 3:9–10: "Do not lie to each other, *since you have taken off your old self with its practices and have put on the new self, which is being renewed in knowledge in the image of its Creator*" (NIV, emphasis added). This teaching from Paul means the way we treat other people completely changes because of Jesus. We get a "new self" that compels us to extend ourselves in love where we might have been tempted to keep to ourselves. We embody the image of our Creator most fully when we look beyond our own self-interest.

I had been wondering why I was struggling to find opportunities to love and serve people; why I felt so lonely moving through the world with two small kids; and how difficult it was to build community. When I gave up the convenience of the self-checkout line, I found it easier to see the image of God in the people around me. If we learn to look around with the love of Christ, I think we will see that purpose and connection are within our grasp after all.

Lord,
Teach me to look around. Teach me to be curious and concerned for others—for their stories, their needs, their pain, and their joy. Help me move through the world the way You did, with my eyes on opportunities to show Your love. Transforming into Your likeness means seeing Your image in others and responding accordingly. Help me, God, to love like You.
Amen.

PART 2

Wisdom + Humility

As a naturally curious person, I find myself looking up random topics on the internet all the time. Widespread access to knowledge can be a gift, but there's also a more insidious side to that kind of instant access. If you're anything like me, I've developed an inflated sense of my own wisdom just because I have a device in my hands. And with my ever-growing awareness and endless supply of information, I'm also growing in anxiety. Maybe you can relate.

Over the next ten days, we will identify ways we try to be wise in our own eyes and how this phenomenon is spinning us out into worry and fear. We'll also explore what it looks like to honor *God's* wisdom and set reasonable expectations for ourselves (when it comes to the limits of our human understanding) so that we can find peace in our hearts and newfound purpose with our lives.

Set your eyes on His calling to humility, and learn to live a life that's focused and submitted to the wisdom of God.

> My heart is not proud, LORD,
> my eyes are not haughty;
> *I do not concern myself with great matters*
> *or things too wonderful for me.*
> *But I have calmed and quieted myself,*
> *I am like a weaned child with its mother;*
> *like a weaned child I am content.*
> *Israel, put your hope in the* LORD
> *both now and forevermore.*
>
> **Psalm 131:1–3 NIV, emphasis added**

We continually ask God to fill you with the knowledge of his will through all the wisdom and understanding that the Spirit gives, so that you may live a life worthy of the Lord and please him in every way.

Colossians 1:9–10 NIV

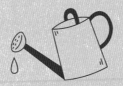

THE STRUGGLES YOU ARE
DEALING WITH ARE
OPPORTUNITIES TO GROW
INTO WHOLENESS.

Prayers of Wisdom

I can remember hundreds of nights in my child-hood bedroom, lying wide awake in my bed, the troubles and conflicts of the day racing through my mind. I have always been prone to self-doubt; I would replay scene after scene of what happened that day, anxiously questioning if I had done the right thing. I would pray equally anxious prayers: "God, I really tried to do the right thing! Please don't be mad at me!"

There were people in my life who were going through hard things.

There were strangers around me who (probably) didn't know Jesus.

I would lay there, wondering how to provide a perfect Christian response to these difficult circumstances, fearing God would be disappointed in me if I did not figure out what to say to these people. I lost so much sleep trying to figure out how I could make God happy, how I could do enough to keep Him from being mad at me.

Looking back, I am so heartbroken for that little girl who believed, to the point of insomnia, that following God was part performance review and part guessing game. These were the prayers of a tender heart that desperately needed true wisdom.

I wish I could share James 1:5 with eight-year-old me, but since I can't, I will share it with you: "If any of you lacks wisdom, you should ask God, who gives generously to all without finding fault, and it will be given to you" (NIV).

How often do we stress and languish and fret over things we can't control, when we could be turning those things over to God in an earnest request for His wisdom? How often do we ask God to answer specific questions or resolve certain situations, instead of asking Him to grow the wisdom required within us?

Of course, God can and will intervene in our lives when we need Him. I'm just suggesting that, perhaps, when we find ourselves spiraling—whether over circumstances we can't control or big decisions that have paralyzed us or even mistakes we have made—maybe part of God's will is that we not only seek solutions, but that we seek to grow in wisdom.

In fact, let's rewind a bit to James 1:2–4: "Consider it pure joy, my brothers and sisters, whenever you face trials of many kinds, because you know that the testing of your faith produces perseverance. Let perseverance finish its work so that you may be mature and complete, not lacking anything" (NIV). Right after this, God generously promises to grant us wisdom.

The struggles you are dealing with? They are opportunities to grow into wholeness. Everything that tests your faith is an opportunity to lean into the wisdom of God. And in order for trials to ultimately produce maturity, God invites us to ask Him for—you guessed it—wisdom!

God delights in the heart that seeks wisdom. When God appeared to Solomon and said he could ask Him anything, you know what Solomon asked for? "An understanding mind to govern your people, that I may discern between good and evil" (1 Kings 3:9 ESV). Because Solomon didn't ask for anything material or self-serving, God was so pleased that He honored this request, and He also granted him riches and long life. We know Solomon as the wisest man who ever lived (1 Kings 4:29–34).

Little Whitney, crying herself to sleep, did not believe that she could ever obtain wisdom, and she did not believe that God loved her enough to give wisdom to her.

Solomon knew he was not wise but went to God with humility. And because of that, God answered his prayer and added heaps of blessings on top of that.

You can spin and struggle and beg God to give you the answer. He certainly could, and He certainly has in the past. But what if God wants to grow your wisdom so that you can stop spinning and struggling? What if God wants you to see the value of wisdom and ask Him for it? What if you looked up from your anxious thoughts and let God bring you into maturity? *What if?*

Lord,
I desire wisdom, and I know You want
to give it. I am tired of anxiously replaying
the events of the day and agonizing over
the right decisions to make. Help me
see these challenges as opportunities to
grow into all You've created me to be.
Amen.

1 2

Submitting to Sovereignty

After graduating from college, I spent a lot of time in prayer trying to discern my career path. Because of my love of embodied theology, I was drawn to nutritional science and dietetics and decided to embark on a journey to be a registered dietitian (RD).

I immediately enrolled in prerequisites and scheduled meetings with the director of the program I intended to join. I commuted forty-five minutes to two different college campuses to complete organic chemistry, biochemistry, and human anatomy classes, which I needed to pass before I could start my program. After a lot of hard work, meticulous planning, and prayer, I got into the RD program!

Fast-forward to the first day of class. I had driven an hour and a half in Southern California traffic, only to spend forty-five more minutes looking for parking. I went to meet with the program director, who told me they had changed the course catalogue. The

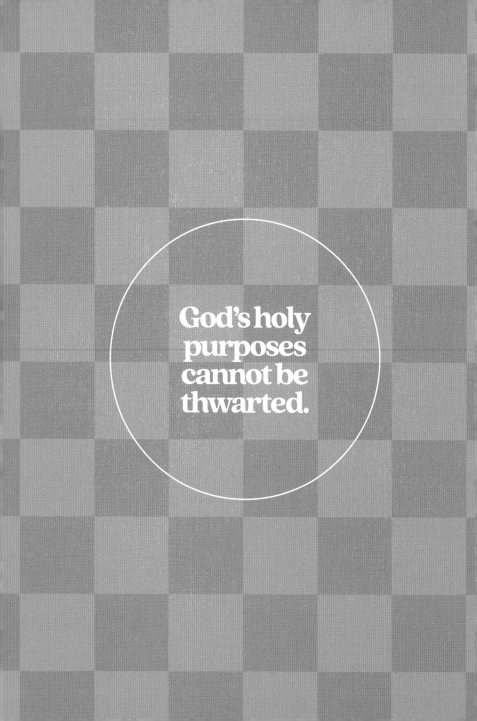

God's holy
purposes
cannot be
thwarted.

two-year program would now take me three. "Oh, and I forgot to tell you: we won't be able to accept the biochemistry course you took. The one we offer will be available next fall." This would add yet another year of coursework.

I'm sorry, what? I couldn't afford two more *years* of school and waste time retaking the prerequisite. I had done all the work and asked all the right questions, and all along, God had opened doors. *What was going on?*

I set aside a whole day crying and venting to God about my confusion, my crumbling career path, and my embarrassment. I remember a lot of silence, except for one tiny nudge from the Holy Spirit: "Stay in this space."

So I just did that. I kept my eyes out for jobs in the wellness industry and, long story short, ended up working as a content manager for a fitness influencer. There, I learned how to impact people through social media and create meaningful content. By the time I left that role, I knew God was calling me to use my newfound expertise in social media to reach and encourage women with biblical truths, which also allowed me to use my bachelor's degree in religious studies. Now I am writing a book, thanking the Lord for leading me into this career that I never would have dreamt of for myself.

It was a weird, frustrating route, but God upended my good plans to get me to His great ones. I prayed thousands of prayers, asking Him to show me the next step, lamenting my failed plans, and telling Him of my doubt.

Prayer isn't submitting our requests to God, waiting for Him to follow our instructions. Prayer is submitting *ourselves*, trusting in the character of God.

"I know that you can do all things;
no purpose of yours can be thwarted.
You asked, 'Who is this that obscures my plans
without knowledge?'
Surely I spoke of things I did not understand,
things too wonderful for me to know."

Job 42:2–3 NIV

If Job, after all that he went through, could still say this of God, then I think it's safe to say we, too, can cling to this truth amid unpredictable change.

God's holy purposes cannot be thwarted. The twists and the turns, the good and the bad—they're coming either way. The sooner we surrender our desire to call the shots in favor of trusting in the sovereignty of a kind, creative God, the sooner we can release our worry, and the more joy we get to experience.

So is it wrong to dream and set big goals? Of course not! But never let those things block your view of what God may have in store for you, the plans that may be outside your scope of vision. You don't have the full picture, and you were never meant to.

Set your eyes on God. Trust that the One who knows the beginning and the ending of the universe is capable of setting your life on the right track. Delight in His faithfulness, and He will give you the desires of your heart, though as you can see from my life, I can't promise those desires will unfold in the way you've planned!

Dear Lord,
I confess that my heart often doubts Your
plans. I confess that I often want to be the writer
of my story, and I want to know my destination
right now. I surrender to Your sovereignty,
God. Take my eyes off my plans and all the
ways I try to force them, and set my eyes on
Your kindness. You have good things for me.
Amen.

Hope for Fools

"**What?** She really thought she could get away with charging eighty dollars for *that*?!" I exclaimed.

Friends, I was in deep. Here I was, using my precious last hour of the day scrolling through the latest drama on CakeTok, the baking community on TikTok. (Important context: I don't even bake.) I had just watched forty-five minutes of a professional cake decorator shaming an unhappy client. I was on the cake decorator's side, until she showed us the cake that started this controversy. And in the kindest of terms, *yikes*.

I jumped to the comment section to see how others reacted. Sure enough, commentor after commentor echoed the same sentiment—that baker's work was astronomically overpriced.

Then, things got personal. "Her ego is way too big." "Her cakes are so bad I thought her account was a joke." "She is disgusting."

I rose from the phone, bleary-eyed and disoriented. How did I get here? Why was this drama so interesting to me?

My scroll through the comments illuminated a problem: because of the dynamics around modern news media, social media, and the availability of information, we believe we are wise enough to judge anything and everything. Because we can search Google or YouTube for the answer to nearly any question, we struggle to believe that comprehensive understanding could be outside our grasp. Whether it looks like taking sides in random internet drama (*à la* CakeTok), or our outrage about complex political issues, we are a culture of quickly rendered, inflexible conclusions.

I've even found myself losing my patience with true, slow learning—especially the part that requires me to sit under the teaching of experts who have dedicated their lives to a particular field. Sitting is boring. I much prefer to get the gist of an issue from the fastest source—and to sound off my opinion just as quickly.

Yet I know myself to be limited in my perspective, right? I'm sure you can think of a time when you made a knee-jerk decision that had an unfortunate impact on your life. If we can't always discern what's right for our own lives—where we have the most context and detail—why would we assume we could have an accurate grasp of reality 100 percent of the time?

Reading Proverbs 26:12 should slow us all down: "Do you see a person wise in their own eyes? There is more hope for a fool than for them" (NIV). To me, this means whenever I find myself feeling like the smartest person in the room (or in the comments section), it's time to take a long, hard pause.

Ultimately, we don't know everything about anything. We need a regular reality check about the limitations of our own understanding.

"For my thoughts are not your thoughts,
neither are your ways my ways," declares the LORD.
"As the heavens are higher than the earth,
so are my ways higher than your ways,
and my thoughts than your thoughts."

Isaiah 55:8–9 NIV

Just like we have not been made to contain all the information in the world, we have not been created to understand the complexity of everything in the world. I think this is a big part of why we are commanded so many times not to judge (Matthew 7:1–5). It's not that we don't know what truth is; it's that our ability to discern the motives of others and to understand all factors in a given situation is often limited. After all, as we read in Proverbs 17:28: "Even a fool who keeps silent is considered wise; when he closes his lips, he is deemed intelligent" (ESV). Perhaps, like me, you need to read that again (don't worry, I'll ask you to at the end of this devotion).

So many of us are trying to sound informed and knowledgeable. So many of us think we have a better grasp on complex topics (and people) than we actually do. We feel pressure to be an expert on everything and experience anxiety when we aren't. We need to remember that the more we try to *look* wise, the more we end up revealing our lack of true understanding.

It's okay not to know it all.

Lord,

I am tired of the constant pressure to pretend I know what is right in all situations, and I'm tired of the way that pressure makes me judge other people. Your ways are higher, and Your thoughts are better. Help me develop an accurate sense of my own wisdom. Help me take my gaze off the futile practice of arbitrating truth and judgment.

Amen.

Hermeneutic
of Humility

Planning vacations for a luxury travel company has been my day job for the past few years. I work hard to curate the best vacation experience for visitors who come to my town. As a local, I have a pretty good sense of the new hot spots and the best locations for photo ops. I know which restaurants have great food and service. I love using my expertise to help people make amazing memories with their loved ones.

Recently, one of my clients sent me a long email of places they wanted to see during their vacation, sourced from random websites. The list included far-flung spots, many of them an hour (or more!) from their accommodations. Almost none of them were on my list of tried-and-true recommendations, most of which were just minutes away.

Working with this client was challenging. Not only were they resistant to my professional expertise, but they wanted me to magically become a local expert for other places where I did

If our lives truly belong to God, then we get to confess that we don't have it all figured out.

not live. I tried to convince them that their initial ideas weren't best suited for their vacation goals, and in the end, I did my best to honor their requests and research good recommendations for their desired day trips. But in the end, their vacation suffered. They complained that they did not experience enough of the local culture, and that they were tired of driving (insert me, eye twitching).

Unfortunately, this client's arrogance cost them. If only they had understood that my lived experience would help them more than their internet searches, they might have had an amazing vacation full of "locals-only" experiences and remember-forever moments right outside their door. A drop of humility might've given them hours of joy back into their vacation.

Humility is the key to moving through our complicated world with joy. First Corinthians 3:18–19 speaks to this: "Do not deceive yourselves. If any of you think you are wise by the standards of this age, you should become 'fools' so that you may become wise. For the wisdom of this world is foolishness in God's sight" (NIV).

If you, like my client, are convinced that you know all you need to render a judgment (whether of travel plans or of another person or situation), you might need to "become a fool." If we want to be wise, we must learn to hold our conclusions with open hands before the Lord.

I hear you asking me something: "So does that mean we should just stop pursuing truth?" Absolutely not! Holding our conclusions loosely simply means that we take our conclusions to God, first through prayer and connection to Christ and *then* through a humble effort to empathize, learn, and research. Jesus is the best at nurturing compassion, kindness, gentleness, and honesty in us when we bring Him into the process.

If God is the preeminent expert in truth, why wouldn't we want Him to be the one helping us navigate complex issues? What's so cool about this is that He is also the originator of all love. When we look to Him, our conclusions are formed by the ultimate wisdom and the kind of love that left heaven to save us.

If our lives truly belong to God, then we get to confess that we don't have it all figured out. If we insist that our positions aren't vulnerable to criticism, we set our wisdom above God's wisdom— which is idolatry.

Maybe it's early in the morning and you have your warm mug of coffee and were just hoping for a sweet, lighthearted reading before you start your day. I'm sorry I spoiled that for you. But I believe that embracing humility is the way to find more joy and less anxiety. We don't need to have all the answers. The more puffed up we get about being right, the easier it is for the Enemy to derail us when we're wrong.

So stay as close to Jesus as you possibly can. When you submit your limited knowledge to His limitless wisdom, you will find true understanding, along with rest and joy growing organically in your life. Retrain your eyes to look at God and His perfect wisdom over and above your own.

God,

I want Your perfect wisdom and not my feeble attempts at truth. Trying to be an expert in everything is stealing my joy. The pressure to judge everything according to my own knowledge has made me both prideful and harsh. I want to move through the world with humility, remembering that I may not know all the answers. Help me set my eyes on Your perfect wisdom and the leading of Your Spirit.

Amen.

How to Test Spirits

When I went to college for religious studies, I heard the same thing constantly: "Don't lose your faith studying theology!" I found it endlessly annoying.

But I nearly did lose my faith while studying the things of God (Mom, if you're reading this, don't say you told me so!). My degree required extensive coursework on world religions, church history, theology, and Christian doctrine. You would think that all of this study would amount to a stronger faith, especially at a Christian school! But for me, it became hard to believe in anything.

I learned about the divisiveness and violence in church history across centuries. I discovered how much of my faith was influenced by the trappings of American culture and began to question some of my influences. In learning about early church councils, I wrestled with how the church ultimately decided upon its central doctrines, like the attributes of the Trinity. The faith I was once so sure about suddenly felt wobbly under my feet, and I froze—unsure of everything and unable to act on anything.

CYNICISM IS SO AFRAID

TO GRAB ONTO SOMETHING

THAT WON'T HOLD

THAT IT NEVER HOLDS ONTO

ANYTHING AT ALL.

Instead of talking to the Lord about my doubt and confusion, I clung to cynicism because cynicism made me feel smart. I became judgmental and dismissive of Christians who were confident in their faith, as if they just weren't smart enough to see all the problems like I could.

According to Oxford Languages, *cynicism* is both the assumption of negative motives and the "inclination to question if something is worthwhile." It both assumes the worst of others and decides that the work of discovery isn't worth it. Cynicism is defensive, an attempt to protect ourselves from the pain of being wrong. It masquerades as education, authority, and wisdom. But cynicism and wisdom are not the same.

First John 4:1–3 can help us tell the difference: "Dear friends, do not believe every spirit, but test the spirits to see whether they are from God, because many false prophets have gone out into the world. This is how you can recognize the Spirit of God: Every spirit that acknowledges that Jesus Christ has come in the flesh is from God, but every spirit that does not acknowledge Jesus is not from God" (NIV).

See? We are not supposed to run from hard questions; we are meant to press into them. John was writing to a community of early Christians who were struggling with division around challenges to key doctrine about the identity of Jesus. Where we might expect one of Jesus' closest friends to get defensive and cynical, John exhorts believers to adopt a posture of openness: *listen, process, respond*. John knows that the truth of Christ will prevail, so he invites his fellow believers into the mystery to find out for themselves.

Wisdom tests everything, and cynicism finds honest testing to be a waste of time. Cynicism is so afraid to grab onto something that won't hold that it never holds onto anything at all.

If Jesus is truly alive, and if the Holy Spirit resides within us, then we are safe to face our doubts and concerns. We know that we have a Guide who will help us as we test the spirits and then do something constructive with what we learn. God can work through the hard questions with us.

I am not saying that we shouldn't point out error in the church. Cynicism and acknowledging problems are two very different things. The former says, "I don't like it, so there is no hope." The latter says, "I don't like it, but we can do something good here." God will always be the best at seeing shortcomings and flaws, yet He never grows cynical. Proverbs 9:10 says, "The fear of the Lord is the beginning of wisdom" (NIV), so we can trust that genuine wisdom will be framed by *both* honesty and hope.

If we are to navigate the mass cynicism in our culture that's contributing to our anxiety and hopelessness, we have to first stop looking to the self-proclaimed experts who only see shortcomings and never see hope. We have to continually pry our eyes away from fake wisdom and instead cast our eyes on Jesus, the wellspring of the hope we crave.

Lord,

Finding the bad in everything has made
me ineffective. I am so tired of being critical
of other people and of myself. Trying to look
wise has had the reverse effect, where now I
even struggle to trust You. I need You to reset
my vision. I need to look away from all that is
wrong, and look instead to You. Help me, God.

Amen.

16

Peace-Loving Wisdom

As the political news cycle became particularly polarizing over the past few years, my husband Tanner and I started questioning some ideologies by which we were raised. He had just finished his master's degree at seminary, and we had just lived through the election of 2016. Despite our questions, we maintained a deep desire to see our family, our friends, and the church remain united on essential doctrine, even when some of the politics got messy. We felt that our changing views were motivated by faithfulness to the words of Jesus and obedience to the Bible, but navigating conversations wisely amid disagreement can be difficult.

For instance, I have a friend who is extremely intelligent and equally outspoken (even aggressive) in their critique of the church. This friend uses big academic words to articulate social problems, and to call for policy changes they believe will right the wrongs in the world. Yet I can't remember a time I saw this person physically interacting with the marginalized communities they often discuss at a distance.

Then there are people like my mother-in-law (hi, Dawn!), who could not care less about academic language and winning the culture-war debates. We don't always agree, but there is no one I see serving and loving people (including those who would call her worldview hateful) on a more regular basis. She is regularly uncomfortable for the sake of others' good.

In presenting these two examples, I am not intending to make a statement about which political views are better. These scenarios could be flipped, and my point would stay the same: worldly wisdom and an impressive academic record do not automatically translate to meaningful action. As important as it is to make well-informed opinions, it's perhaps even more crucial to bear the fruit of the Spirit.

So how can we make sure that our wisdom leads to meaningful action? How can we make sure that the wisdom we are living by is the godly kind of wisdom?

Glad you asked. Let's look at James 3.

"Who is wise and understanding among you? Let them show it by their good life, by deeds done in the humility that comes from wisdom. . . . But the wisdom that comes from heaven is first of all pure; then peace-loving, considerate, submissive, full of mercy and good fruit, impartial and sincere. Peacemakers who sow in peace reap a harvest of righteousness" (13, 17–18 NIV).

Real wisdom from God results in humility, and that humility bears good deeds.

Real wisdom is not hurling the better clap back or the smarter take; real wisdom is lived.

The first way to test whether your wisdom is godly is to assess the tone of your life. Do your ideas come with a strong side of cynicism? Do rage, fear, contempt, and pride frame all your opinions? Then I think it's safe to say that your wisdom is not aligned with God's wisdom. Do your convictions translate to deeds done in humility and peacemaking? If not, James might've suggested that your convictions are likely not rooted in God's wisdom.

I share this not to ignite a political discussion. I share this because the time we live in brings much confusion and much emotion about who is right and who is wrong.

Maybe, in our quest for wisdom, it's time we start looking for its fruit. James has told us point-blank what real wisdom will look like. If you want to be wise, watch the people who are loving and serving real people in real ways. When you are doing your best to look people in the eye and love them, your ideology doesn't always matter as much as you think it will.

Look for the wisdom that lives a good life of service. Look for the people who are pushing outside of their comfort zones, not just to say hard things, but to do hard things for hard people (whomever that may be for them). Look for lovers of peace—those who are considerate and overflowing with mercy. Look for people who don't play favorites and who put their whole heart in. Look at the fruit.

Lord,
When I feel overwhelmed by all the cynicism
and all the people claiming to be wise, help me
look at their fruit to discern whether what they're
saying is worth listening to. I pray that Your Holy
Spirit would guide me to Your truth and Your
wisdom, and that through it all, You would keep
my heart humble. Grow in me a love of peace.
Help me set my eyes on the fruit of true wisdom.
Amen.

17

Wisdom in Community

I have done a lot of high school ministry in the form of camp counseling, small group leading, mentoring, and coffee dates over the past ten years. And in the words of Regina George's mom in *Mean Girls*, "You girls keep me young, I love you so much." Recently, I have observed a shift in how younger generations speak about themselves. When I was in high school, I didn't hear many girls talk about their diagnosed depression or generalized anxiety disorder or being on the autism spectrum. The language and awareness that young people have around mental health has skyrocketed in sophistication in the past few years.

Social media gets much of the credit for this shift, and that comes with pros and cons. The major pro is the destigmatization of mental health issues and the availability of resources surrounding them. One big con is that in the process of becoming more educated, it has become too easy for young people with zero professional training to self-diagnose any number of mental health

Don't
Spiral
Alone.

disorders in total isolation based on information they get from the internet.

An important note: I am not casting doubt on any diagnosis. I am not denying that social media can be a powerful tool for mental health awareness. I am simply commenting on the phenomenon of self-diagnosis that many experts have also acknowledged in recent years.

This is tricky territory, so I will focus on my own experience. I saw a video about ADHD in high-achieving women, and I was *convinced* that I had it. The algorithm picked up on my interest and showed me more content around this topic (which only made my anxiety worse!). I thought this diagnosis explained my issues with friendships, my struggles to keep my car clean, and why I remember nothing from high school! To me, self-diagnosing myself as having ADHD felt like a silver bullet to explain my biggest struggles and a lingering sense of discomfort with myself.

Here's the thing though: I *don't* have ADHD. Because I was researching this complex condition all by myself on the internet, the details that resonated with me jumped off the page, and the ones that didn't, I glazed over. My misdiagnosis, which I came to by myself, resulted in more confusion and frustration than before.

We all want to know why we feel so out of place, lonely, and awkward. *Any* diagnosis would be a relief! For me, trying to solve my existential discomfort armed with nothing but my own anxieties and a smartphone only served to isolate me further.

If you're self-diagnosing a physical or mental health issue and stirring up anxiety in your soul, I encourage you to seek out professional help. Don't rob yourself of the care that can improve your life! Invite loved ones into the conversation. Don't spiral alone.

I am of the firm belief that Jesus cares deeply about our health—mental, physical, and relational. He designed you to need others, and we are blessed to be living in a time with professionals who are more equipped than ever before to diagnose and treat our ailments.

The Bible teaches us that we can cast our anxieties upon Him because He cares about us (1 Peter 5:7). We don't have to conceal our problems or try to wish them away. We can give Him our unknowns, including our mental health struggles and other struggles that we don't know how to name. He has given us the common grace of therapists and treatments if we need a little extra help managing what's weighing so heavily upon us.

That pervasive sense of worry that just takes over sometimes? I have been there. I need Him most in those moments. The deep sadness or embarrassment that sometimes makes it hard to reach out to others? You are not weird or broken. I feel it too.

Jesus wants you to invite trusted individuals into your pain and remember, even in the dark moments, you were made *good*. He is beckoning you to stop fixating on the overwhelming litany of things that could be wrong and to instead look at the people He has placed in your life to walk with you through your struggles. Sometimes, letting other people into our pain is the best way to let God in too.

Dear God,
I look around and see so many possibilities
of what's wrong with me, so many explanations
for why I am struggling. Please meet me
in this confusion and help me see clearly.
Please help me let others in and to trust that
You will bring light through Your people.
Amen.

Expectations Are Everything

I had my son, Judah, in 2020. I found out I was pregnant right as the world went into lockdown and gave birth during one of the most severe peaks of the pandemic in California. I went to most of my doctor's appointments alone. As we invited our first child into the world, I needed to be surrounded by community. But I was forced into isolation, left mostly to the internet to help me prepare.

Then, just like that, I was holding my newborn, totally in love. Yet almost immediately, I became terrified by the notion that anything bad could happen to him. I felt desperate. Panic gripped my chest so tightly I could hardly breathe. Stress is normal when you're a parent to a newborn. But I was so raw that even small challenges sent me spiraling. With my doctor's recommendation, I decided to go on medication until my emotions regulated.

Here's the thing though—even with my panic, I was so happy. I could lose myself for hours studying Judah's dimpled hands and holding him while he slept. I loved bringing him on walks to

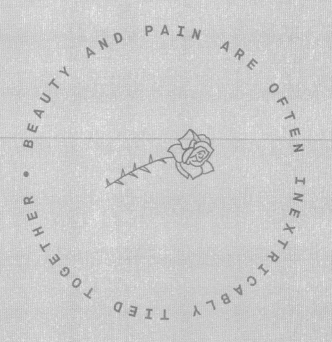

BEAUTY AND PAIN ARE OFTEN INEXTRICABLY TIED TOGETHER • BEAUTY TIED TOGETHER •

watch him take in his new world. I even loved that the pandemic-mandated quarantine granted my husband an extra three months at home with us.

Living in peace means acknowledging that beauty and pain are often inextricably tied together. There is wisdom in holding this tension and knowing that life can be beautiful, even if it's really, really hard. Giving birth was painful, but I've never done anything more profound. Motherhood brought new anxiety into my life, but also one of the deepest loves I have ever known.

Sometimes, beauty hurts. Sometimes, pain can heal.

How can we make peace with pain in this world and still embrace life's joys? Godly wisdom makes space for both.

The intermingling of beauty and pain is a theological concept, sometimes referred to as the "already but not yet." Christ has *already* conquered death, *yet* we are waiting for the complete consummation of this victory when He returns for His people. We know that sickness does not get the final word, yet we still recognize that disease is doing harm. We know that the corruption, racism, exploitation, and glorification of sin are just a long, final scream of death in the grand scheme of eternity, but that knowledge doesn't undo the very legitimate pain of our present.

When we expect to feel at ease in this world, we are setting ourselves up for disappointment, angst, and resentment. We start to think, *God, how could you? God, why me?* But when we correctly understand that God's work is *not yet* complete in the world, we can find peace in times of uncertainty and fear.

Colossians 2:9–10 says, "For in Christ all the fullness of the Deity lives in bodily form, and in Christ you have been brought to fullness" (NIV). Other translations say, "In Him, you have been made complete" (NASB). Well, I don't always feel full. I don't feel complete. That's not because Paul is lying, and it's not because Jesus didn't redeem all things on the cross. No, all of creation (including us!) has already been fully redeemed, and yet we will not see its fullness until Christ returns.

This framework of "already, but not yet" doesn't suggest that you accept your misery and soldier on. No, this framework says that mental illness, physical ailments, and loneliness are to be expected in a broken world, and that God's grace can come in the form of professional help and authentic community. Wisdom, then, invites us into honest and emotional prayer, humbly pleading for God to change our circumstances, but not pridefully demanding it. The key to minimizing our anxiety is calibrating our expectations to living in an imperfect world and asking God to do a merciful work within it and through us. In this world we will have trouble around us and within us. We can rest our eyes from constantly searching for a life without hardship, and instead dig deep into relationships with others, ultimately looking to Christ alone to complete us when He restores all things.

God,

Sometimes I feel incomplete and insufficient.
I have found myself anxiously chasing after
an adversity-free life, even though You never
promised that to me. Help me look to You
in difficult times and become clear-eyed
about facing hardship, knowing that the full
realization of Your victory is yet to come. Help
me rest and find peace in communion with
You and others when my heart feels frantic.

Amen.

19

It's Okay Not to Listen (to Everyone)

Sometimes, wisdom means keeping close watch over the voices you're allowing to speak into your life. Wisdom means knowing who to listen to, and which voices we may need to let fade away.

I was in the gym one morning, doing my best to stay active during my second pregnancy. I was early in my first trimester and hadn't even told my closest friends. There was no bump in sight, but I was so sick and extremely bloated from the pregnancy hormones (and the fact that literally all I could eat was bread). Now, I love seeing other women look absolutely cute when they're working out, but I was squarely in the "huge T-shirt and visibly struggling" camp at this point.

"You should think about lifting heavier!" A tinny, young male voice called out to me from across the room. I had seen this guy around, but we didn't know each other. "The light weights won't really help with building muscle mass," he explained before citing some study he definitely heard about on some podcast. I let it slide; I wasn't about to announce my pregnancy to this rando before my best friends even knew.

Later that week, he was back in his infinite wisdom, explaining how the treadmill "wasn't doing anything for me." I considered throwing up on him, but I thought better of it and said, "Oh, good idea!"

A few days later, he very kindly suggested some ab exercises that would "get real results," as opposed to the planks I was attempting. I said, "Thanks!" and gave it my best shot just to appease him so he would leave.

You know what I learned later? The exercise he suggested is not recommended for pregnant women. My annoyance at the gym guy quickly transformed into shame. *Why would you change your workout to make this guy happy when he doesn't even know you're pregnant?* This person did not deserve influence in my life: he didn't know me, and he didn't know my circumstances.

Have you ever been there, listening to the "wisdom" of people who have no business speaking into your life? My people-pleasing tendencies can lead me to take advice from anyone who offers. I often find my head spinning in confusion from the sheer diversity of opinions I've heard from the people in my life.

It's good and right to tune out some voices when it comes to your personal decision-making. There is wisdom in allowing only a handful of trusted people who know you well and will push you toward the Lord to hold influence over your life. In other words, it's okay to not listen to the proverbial random gym guys roaming around, offering their surface-level opinions about things to which you haven't offered them access.

"Blessed is the one who does not walk in step with the wicked or stand in the way that sinners take or sit in the company of mockers, but whose delight is in the law of the Lord, and who meditates on his law day and night. That person is like a tree planted by streams of water, which yields its fruit in season and whose leaf does not wither—whatever they do prospers" (Psalm 1:1–3 NIV).

**Say it with me:
It's okay not to listen
to everyone.**

We must exercise sharp discernment about which voices we obey. We need to be intentional and wise with whose counsel we allow to guide our choices.

So here's our litmus test for the advice of others:

If they don't know your heart and don't genuinely want you to thrive, think twice before welcoming their "wisdom."

If they don't love the LORD and believe that knowing Him is the highest and best good, they may not be the best source of wisdom for you.

If they don't ask questions before firing off an opinion, proceed with caution.

If the wisdom they give contradicts Scripture, then it isn't true wisdom.

Guard your heart, for your life springs from it. Not everyone should get access, and the people you trust for direction should be trusted, godly people who want your good.

Breathe. Say it with me: It's okay not to listen to everyone.

TODAY'S READING: PSALM 1
FOR ADDITIONAL STUDY: PROVERBS 4

God,
I pray that You would help me discern who is worth listening to, and what wisdom is worth keeping. Help me find people I can trust who will offer sound advice for my good and Your glory. Guard my heart, and teach me how to do it too.
Amen.

Through Many Advisers

In college, I was really sick for about a year. My eyes were bloodshot (literally blood-red), and I got these crazy welts on my legs—about fifty of them—some of which swelled to the size of golf balls. I struggled to sleep. I had near-constant headaches. Needless to say, I looked very, very cute during this chapter of my life (false), and my future husband could not help but to ask me on a date (weirdly true). No one knew what was going on, but some of my symptoms pointed to some very serious conditions, so I was eager for answers.

I made appointments with every specialist imaginable—a rheumatologist, an internist, a renowned infectious disease doctor, another doctor who specialized in complications from parasite exposure, and my childhood pediatrician for good measure, among others. I was fortunate to have good insurance, because otherwise I would have spent thousands of dollars on medical care. By the time I left an appointment, I had yet another suggestion for a doctor who might have the expertise to diagnose my elusive condition.

Doctors are some of the most educated professionals in our society, right? So why did they continue to send me to other doctors with different expertise? These doctors were wise enough to know that a variety of informed opinions was my best bet at success. They were so well-versed in their work that they had the humility to know that sometimes, another expert's voice would be more beneficial. This was true of my medical mystery, and it's true of our lives in general.

When we are deciding whose wisdom to heed, we should seek the expertise of trusted people with diverse backgrounds and experiences that will ultimately render well-rounded, deeply rooted advice. We do well to seek the "experts" who are smart enough to know that their knowledge has limits. While we should indeed exercise discernment in who we allow influence in our lives, we must also strive to glean insight from different perspectives (so long as that insight falls within the parameters explained in the previous devotion).

Humbly exposing ourselves to perspectives we may initially dismiss can often enrich and grow us. In Numbers 22, God used a literal donkey to correct and redirect the prophet Balaam, who was on his way to curse Israel. Now, I would not recommend searching for your next mentor at a livestock auction, but God can clearly use unexpected sources to speak wisdom into our lives.

I want us to have hearts that are open to receive it wherever it may come.

Discerning wisdom doesn't mean you plug your ears to people with different opinions and beliefs; discerning wisdom means listening closely to a range of voices, and then intentionally comparing that insight to the truth of the Bible and to the counsel of the trusted advisers in your life.

The Bible teaches us that "victory is won through many advisers" (Proverbs 11:14 NIV). The more trustworthy advisers we can find, the better off we will be. Why? Many advisers are only helpful if they are bringing different offerings to the table.

There is an inherent tension here. We want to be selective about counsel, yet open enough to receive it. We want to be discerning in who we allow to influence us, yet we don't want to shut our ears to the opinions of people we may not ultimately agree with.

Let me exhort you to press into this tension with prayer and a posture of listening, first to God and then to others. To construct a circle of wise, trusted people from a diversity of backgrounds who also love you and love the Lord is a tall order—I know that. I also believe that if we patiently, prayerfully search for wise counsel (even in unexpected places that pull us out of our comfort zones), God is faithful to provide it. We just need to have the humility to know that we need as much good help as we can get along with the wisdom to continuously return to the Lord as our gauge of truth. As we've been counseled in Proverbs 19:20: "Listen to advice and accept discipline, and at the end you will be counted among the wise" (NIV).

Dear God,
Teach me to listen with both discernment
and humility. Show me where to find wise,
godly voices that also represent a diverse
range of experiences and backgrounds.
Guide me as I seek to surround myself
with many trustworthy advisers.
Amen.

PART 3

Capacity + Burnout

Have you ever known true exhaustion? Even after twelve hours of sleep, you're still fatigued and staring into space. Few of your required activities leave you feeling replenished. You spend the whole day looking forward to its end. And then, when you finally sit down to relax, all you can think about are the things you should be doing instead.

The cycle is unrelenting and unfulfilling. We are always tired, yet never able to turn off our minds and our anxious hearts so we can rest.

The world loves to tell us that we can achieve anything and have it all. These sound like encouragements, but they're damaging lies. We simply are not wired to do everything, nor do we have the capacity to. When we chase after *everything*, we inevitably end up achieving very little. And then we wonder why we're burned out and sad.

Over the next ten days, we're going to explore patterns of where we're trying to do too much, and how we may employ some God-given boundaries and limits to set realistic and effective expectations for ourselves. Only then will we learn to rest in the arms of Jesus and focus our strengths to bring honor and glory to His name and His people.

So set your eyes on God's limitlessness, and surrender to the God-given limits of your own.

> Do you not know? Have you not heard?
> The LORD is the everlasting God, the Creator of the
>   ends of the earth.
> He will not grow tired or weary, and his
>   understanding no one can fathom.
> He gives strength to the weary and increases the
>   power of the weak.
> Even youths grow tired and weary, and young men
>   stumble and fall;
> but those who hope in the LORD will renew their
>   strength.
> They will soar on wings like eagles; they will run
>   and not grow weary,
> They will walk and not be faint.

Isaiah 40:28–31 NIV

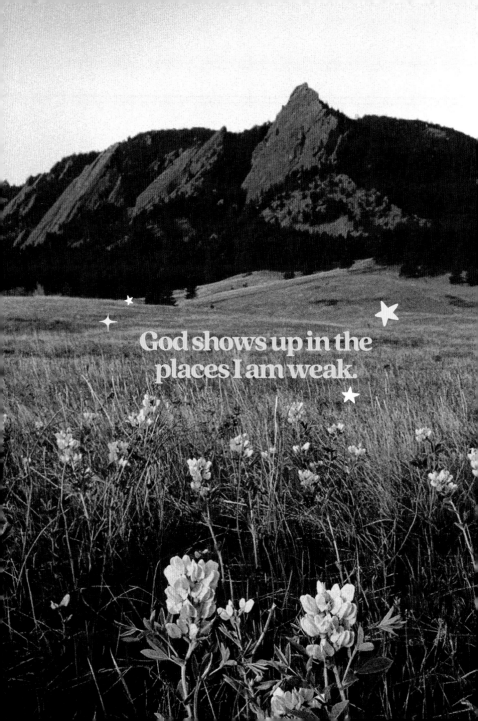

God shows up in the places I am weak.

But a Breath

As I write this, I am on my lunch break from my day job with my work computer open to my email inbox. On the other side of my desk is my baby monitor, toggling between my two-year-old son's room (he's supposed to be napping, but isn't) and my seven-month-old daughter's crib (she's supposed to be napping and actually *is*, praise the Lord). I have my phone open to a conversation about weekend plans that need to get finalized ASAP. Deadlines loom, bills need to be paid, and gifts need to be sent for friends' birthdays. I usually squeeze in housework after the kids are sleeping, or when my babysitter is here. On paper, I am doing it all.

I've cried no less than five times today. Even on the best days, when I am checking off my to-do list, I am swiftly derailed by the smallest change to my plans for the day. Even if I manage to pull off a few "good" days in a row, I am exhausted and burned out by the end of the week. I am learning—down to the marrow of my tired thirty-year-old bones—that I cannot do it all.

And still, I tell myself that I *have* to. Something in me thinks that if I stop achieving, my life and family will fall apart. Some tasks *are* necessary, but I've convinced myself that the success and functioning of my life depends wholly on me. In moments of true exhaustion, I've put too much focus on my own abilities and efficiency and not enough on God's. I have found that a big part of fighting back burnout has been reorienting my perspective (i.e., setting my eyes higher, if you will).

Yes, the work must get done. But if I drop a ball, I can find rest knowing God is still God. If I forget to pay a bill, for example, everything will still be okay! God will continue to provide for our family.

When I'm weary and needing a break, God shows up in the places I am weak. I may not feel like a fun mom all the time, but I have seen God provide me with a miraculous burst of energy on the days when I am at my limit. When I feel like I will never sleep again, God is faithful to replenish me. I've had friends show up with coffee unannounced on days I've been struggling; I've had appointments inexplicably cancelled on days I am losing it. God is still taking care of me, even in the smallest ways.

Ultimately, when we're feeling depleted, it's good to remember that God is God. He is capable of juggling an infinite number of tasks. He directs the course of history. He is in control—not me.

When we rightly understand that every good thing does not depend on us—but rather on Him—the burden of our to-do list lifts. Even on these crazy long days (unavoidable as they may be in some seasons), can we cling to the fact that all of our work is perhaps a form of worship? Like Paul told the Colossians, "Whatever you do, work at it with all your heart, as working for the Lord, not for human masters, since you know that you will receive an inheritance from the Lord as a reward. It is the Lord Christ you are serving" (Colossians 3:23–24 NIV).

We do the work as best we can with whatever we have to offer, meager as it may seem some days. Then, we trust that Jesus is gracious and powerful enough to use what we have to sustain us in our weakness, so long as our hearts are postured toward His sufficiency and not our own.

My schedule is insane right now. That may be the case for a little while longer, and I imagine the same may be true for you today. I'm *not* going to reassure you that we can do it all. What I *will* do is remind you that Jesus makes these long days matter when we surrender the striving. Look up. He's got you.

Lord,

Give me the grace to remember that my
peace does not depend on my ability to get
things done or achieve big wins. I invite You
into my long list of responsibilities and ask
You to stand in for me in the places where I
am lacking today. Remind me that my days are
short, and that eternal work belongs to You
alone. Remind me that all of this is just worship.
I am tired, God, and I want to lean on You.

Amen.

22

Dependence Is the Sweet Spot

I talk to a lot of college and high school girls, and many of them want to know what it's like having a baby. My answer is: motherhood is my favorite thing, but it's ruined my rhythms. Naps, for example: Did you know that if a baby is awake for too long, they can get so tired that they become unable to sleep? But if you *don't* keep them up long enough, they're also not able to sleep? I knew having a baby would be hard, but I did not account for the mental energy I would use just trying to calculate when my baby would nap.

There's this magical sweet spot where, I am told, babies are sleepy but not *too* sleepy, and you can lay them down with minimal drama for a nice, long nap. If that has been your experience with baby naps, I very much love that for you. But at this time, I am asking that you respect my mental health and not tell me about it. Thank you so much.

We do
our best
and then
we rest.

I've been trying to do everything perfectly to get my daughter, Thea, to sleep long enough for me to get anything done, and it just isn't working. I have even found myself feeling anger toward my tiny baby for not sleeping (which, on paper, sounds ridiculous).

On one particularly frustrating day of bad naps, I finally accepted that I would never be able to control naptime, and I released it to the Lord. And you know what? I found myself feeling more at peace because I wasn't trying to bear a burden that wasn't mine. I also noticed that, somehow, the timing of each day (very dependent on my kids' sleep schedules) miraculously aligned in such a way that I was able to get the essential tasks of the day done. My white-knuckle grip on achieving and engineering and controlling hadn't created one more minute of time, but it did make me miserable.

In these many months worrying and navigating my daughter's sleep habits, God reminded me of one simple fact: I am not in control. Becoming a parent reoriented me to the futility of my own ability. There comes a point when we do our very best and then release our work to God, knowing that ultimately, He alone is in control. This is a beautiful gift: we do our best, and then we rest.

Making an effort to succeed is part of good stewardship. The problem comes when we start to believe that we alone are in control of our days, and that we are the ones wholly responsible for the outcome. We must remember that God is the builder, and we are partnering with Him as He does good work in and through us. "For we are co-workers in God's service; you are God's field, God's building" (1 Corinthians 3:9 NIV).

Psalm 127 puts it this way:

> Unless the LORD builds the house,
> the builders labor in vain.
> Unless the LORD watches over the city,
> the guards stand watch in vain.
> In vain you rise early
> and stay up late,
> toiling for food to eat—
> for he grants sleep to those he loves.
>
> Psalm 127:1–2 NIV

In other words, when it comes to our lives, we want to control the details and know exactly what the end product will look like. But let me assure you: God's way is so much better.

Your very best blueprint pales in comparison to what God wants to do with your life. You can't control every facet of your life, including naptimes and to-do lists, or build the perfect life in your own strength. Surrender your work—the best you've got today, wherever that finds you—to God, trusting that He is a skilled builder. Then, accept the rest He wants to give you. Dependence is the sweet spot, my friend.

Dear God,
Thank You for being the builder. I want
to rest in Your plans for me, and for my work
to spring from trust. I will show up each
day and give You the best I've got, then I will
trust that You are in control. Help my heart
to truly learn the beauty of dependence.
Amen.

Counterfeit Rest

After a long day juggling little kids, corporate work, household chores, and my own basic human needs (wildly luxurious of me to insist upon showering!), nothing sounds better than a night of mindless reality television. The Bachelor franchise has me in a chokehold. Give me the remote and let me critique the edited-beyond-recognition version of what a twenty-two-year-old from San Diego has to say about finding love. Let me get lost in "the most dramatic season in *Bachelor* history" (which is somehow all of them). That show shuts off my brain unlike anything else. I'm not proud of it, but there comes a time when we all must own our truth.

But here's the thing: bingeing reality TV doesn't actually impart lasting peace and renewal. It actually detracts from the sleep I need to function.

My go-to strategy for winding down, then, is not genuine rest. Rest brings restoration, but my late-night TV-bingeing is just a quick hit of dopamine that allows me to escape and numb out for a while. My goal in these moments is to shut down as quickly as possible and disengage with the real world.

What's your preferred form of counterfeit "rest"? Is it online shopping? Gossiping with your best friend? Getting lost in a novel? It could even be a relationship. Maybe it's something you wish I wouldn't bring up, like internet porn or drugs or the glass of wine that turns into four. Your escape doesn't have to be inherently sinful, but it certainly might be. As far as I'm concerned, *anything* we use to numb ourselves is something we need to be aware of.

Just like a good night's sleep, sometimes true rest requires us to put down the devices and the distractions. Rest that restores may counterintuitively require us to step away from our go-to sources of temporary comfort.

In Exodus, God quite literally commanded His people to rest one day each week (Exodus 20:8–11), and there is much to learn from what this divinely ordained rest entailed.

On this Sabbath day, the Israelites were not to carry burdens of any kind (Jeremiah 17:21–22). They were to set down their physical and spiritual burdens as an act of surrender and dependence that flies in the face of modern hustle culture. They were also prohibited from buying and selling (Nehemiah 13:15–17), meaning they were to take a break from commerce. How much more do we, living in this materialism-driven society, need a break from the constant consumerism that draws us in?

In the wilderness, the Israelites were instructed to prepare their manna for the Sabbath a day in advance (Exodus 16:21–30). This was a sign of their reliance on God alone for provision and a surrender of their striving. While we are no longer bound to the Old Testament Sabbath laws, we, too, will benefit from the true rest that comes from intentionally acknowledging that He alone sustains us. Sabbath was intended to take our eyes off the ways of this world and to set them onto God's kingdom.

When we make space to reorient ourselves to the reality of God's power and love, we will find our hearts truly revived. As Romans 12:1–2 says, "Therefore, I urge you, brothers and sisters, in view of God's mercy, to offer your bodies as a living sacrifice, holy and pleasing to God—this is your true and proper worship. Do not conform to the pattern of this world, but be transformed by the renewing of your mind. Then you will be able to test and approve what God's will is—his good, pleasing and perfect will" (NIV).

When we're in need of rest, the last thing we want to do is immerse ourselves *more* deeply into the patterns of this world. Reality TV, drinking, and shopping—really anything that offers the counterfeit rest of escapism—do not retune our hearts to the reality of God's kingdom, nor do they offer the peace and renewal that we find in it.

Your heart needs that kind of true renewal. What "patterns of this world" have you been going to for counterfeit rest? Maybe today is the day to stop settling for "rest" that doesn't truly restore.

Lord,
I desire true, restorative rest for my burned-out heart and my exhausted body. Show me what counterfeits I have been leaning on to escape and numb out. Help me create space to reorient to Your provision and Your kingdom.
In Your mercy, God, renew my mind.
Amen.

IN SLOWING DOWN,

YOU ARE MAKING SPACE

FOR GOD TO RESTORE YOU

BACK TO FULL HEALTH.

Making Space for Solitude

I hate the quiet. I come from a TV-always-on-in-the-background kind of family. Now that everyone and their mother has a podcast, I am constantly listening to commentary on current events, going on a deep dive into some obscure topic, or half-absorbing a sermon. (I have nothing if not range.) Rarely will you find me without one AirPod in my ear, half listening while I go about my day.

Having suffered from anxiety-related insomnia for a long time, I often fall asleep listening to a podcast—something interesting, but not too stimulating. The point is: I like low-grade distraction to keep me from thinking too much. I fear where my mind will go if I'm left to my own thoughts in the silence. Distraction feels safer.

Maybe you're addicted to noise like I am. Perhaps your low-grade distraction depends on your phone and the apps that are engineered to fill your attention. Maybe you're addicted to busyness, packing your calendar so you're never without something to occupy your time. One thing is clear: many of us live in active avoidance of solitude.

As a spiritual discipline, solitude (and the silence that it requires) creates "an open, empty space where we are enabled to become attentive to God" (Foster). Jesus—God incarnate—regularly sought solitude for Himself. During His three-year ministry, Jesus walked hundreds of miles around modern-day Israel and Palestine, healing and preaching to crowds of people—an undoubtedly draining endeavor, like we read about in Luke 8:43–48 as power literally left Jesus as the bleeding woman touched Him. And often, Jesus made intentional effort to "withdr[a]w to lonely places and pray" (Luke 5:16 NIV). He sought solitude after healing others (Mark 1:35). He sought solitude when He grieved John the Baptist's death (Matthew 14:13). He sought solitude as He prepared for His own death (Luke 22:39–44).

Perhaps Jesus would have preferred to stay with His friends. Maybe He, too, would have liked to simply numb out like I often do. Solitude is called a spiritual *discipline*, after all. Jesus knew His work necessitated time alone with His Father. To renew our minds and obtain true rest, we must seek out quiet places where we actually stand a chance of hearing God speak.

In the Old Testament, Moses would withdraw from the Israelite camp to the "tent of meeting," where "the LORD would speak to Moses face to face, as one speaks to a friend" (Exodus 33:11 NIV). On one such occasion, Moses shared his anxieties with God. God's reply was profound and affirms our foundational need to be in quiet places, alone with God: "My Presence will go with you, and I will give you rest" (Exodus 33:14 NIV). In the quiet, God gave Moses clear direction for leading His people. Moses returned to the camp literally glowing (Exodus 34:34–35) and renewed to lead a whole community of people who relied upon him.

Maybe you're afraid of solitude like I am. Maybe you fear what you'll hear in the quiet, or the lies that seem louder when you're undistracted. Maybe you suspect that if you slow down for even one hour, you could flame out completely, with no hope of rekindling your fire.

Let me give you courage: When you choose to spend time in solitude, what you're really choosing is closeness to a good Father who is pleased with you. When you choose to spend time in silence, you're choosing to amplify His voice above all others. When you choose to slow down, you are making space for God to restore you back to full health.

Solitude isn't scary. Solitude is the safest thing we can do.

Trade your counterfeit rest for the renewal that comes from solitude—even if, at first, you struggle. Make yourself a cup of coffee and find a cozy chair to tuck into while you pour out your heart to your Father. Go for a walk at sunset, leaving your headphones behind. I can't wait for you to hear what the still, small voice of God has been trying to tell you. I can't wait for you to experience the true rest that solitude has been offering you all this time.

Draw near to God, and He will draw near to you.

Father,
Solitude is scary, but I want to draw near
to You. I want to find the true rest that comes
from a close, real relationship with You. Give
me the courage to be alone in the quiet; help me
experience the rest that comes from solitude.
Amen.

25

Not My Job

Julia was dating a guy at our church, and for a whole summer she attended almost every event we had. She was quirky, with pink streaks in her hair, an affinity for anime, and big issues with many Christian beliefs and evangelical culture.

I liked Julia; she was always respectful. She wasn't much of a talker, but I was confident if I dedicated enough time to conversation with her, she would come around. I was determined to prove to her that Christians aren't so bad after all! She would see how real the love of Christ was in our community (and of course, in me). She would receive the gospel and reform her life, and we would all ride off into the sunset! I had a plan to change Julia, and I couldn't wait to get started.

On the annual summer trip for the church college group (of which my husband was the pastor), we paired the students with prayer partners. This often leads to deeper friendships, with heart-to-heart talks extending late into the night. Mature Christian pastor's wife that I was, I decided that I would be Julia's prayer partner. She needed me, after all.

The first night, we were out on the deck of our cabin, looking up at the stars from our Adirondack chairs. I asked Julia to tell me her life story. I *knew* that if we bonded, I could make a difference in her life.

"Um, I grew up in California, and my parents are divorced. What else do you want to know?" Julia replied, totally deadpan.

I tried again. "Well, like, what has been your biggest struggle?"

"Dumb people," Julia quipped. She did not appear to be interested in bonding with me.

I laughed nervously.

"Okay, good talk! Do we have to pray now?" Julia said after she had already stood up and gathered her things.

Of course, I didn't force her to pray with me. While I watched her walk back into the cabin, I felt shame and even a little anger. *What is wrong with me? I am a failure of a Christian.*

I'd love to say that we turned a corner the following nights, but no. At best, we would chitchat aimlessly before we parted ways. I found myself increasingly stressed over the state of her soul. My efforts were well-meaning but doomed to fail. I wasn't just trying to change her mind about Christianity. I was trying to change *her*.

Here's the truth: human beings can't change hearts. When I take on the changing of human hearts as my job—*my* responsibility—I set myself up for discouragement and burnout. It will never work.

God alone brings about change in human hearts through His Spirit (Ezekiel 36:26–27). He alone can save. What is our job then? How do we partner with God as He changes hearts? Great question! Paul has an answer:

The harder you
try to do a job
that only God
can, the more
burned out you
will become.

"Therefore, if anyone is in Christ, the new creation has come: The old has gone, the new is here! All this is from God, who reconciled us to himself through Christ and gave us the ministry of reconciliation: that God was reconciling the world to himself in Christ, not counting people's sins against them. And he has committed to us the message of reconciliation. We are therefore Christ's ambassadors, as though God were making his appeal through us" (2 Corinthians 5:17–20 NIV).

God redeemed us to the ministry of reconciliation, not the ministry of heart makeovers or behavior overhauls. We love people with sincerity, with a genuine desire for their good. We serve people joyfully, without strings or conditions attached. We live as renewed people, we tell of what God has done, and we wait for God to change people's hearts.

If God isn't counting people's sins against them, far be it from me to take personal offense when people don't change in the way I think they should.

We cannot change people. The harder you try to do a job that only God can, the more burned out you will become. World change in God's kingdom rarely looks the way we think it should; it starts in humble places with gentle hearts amid wholehearted dependence. You, my friend, are a terrible changer of people, but you make an *amazing* ambassador for God's kingdom. Do your job and trust God will do His.

Lord,
I am sorry when I try to exact power that is only Yours to wield. Thank You that heart change is not my job, and thank You for the honor of representing You in the world. Shift my gaze to Your power and off my own so I can do kingdom work with You.
Amen.

PRAYER CORRECTED
MY BELIEFS ABOUT MY OWN
CAPACITY AND RENEWED
MY ENERGY.

26

Fix You

I am a classic oldest sister. I am so used to being followed that when others don't follow my lead, I find it disorienting. The same is true of the advice I give to others. I find it difficult to remain cool when people ask for my advice and do not follow it. No one knows this better than my younger sister, Haley. I do not hold my tongue when I think she's chosen the wrong shoes or overdone it on her eyebrows. I've also spoken up, loudly, when I thought she had room to grow spiritually.

During a particularly tough season of her life, I was quick to offer my blueprint for fixing her life. When she didn't follow my instructions, I would initiate more conversations about how I felt she was falling short, and I was waiting for her to get with my program. The more I shamed and chastised her, the more she withdrew from me. She stopped giving me access to the parts of her life that I insisted on condemning. My attempts to help were unsuccessful and only caused further discouragement and disruption in our relationship. I felt like a failure.

I became so tired of trying to help her. Amid my burnout, I

tried something wild: I started praying. And you know what? The more I prayed for her, the more I genuinely desired that she would flourish. My anxiety dissipated, trusting that God was at work in my sister's life. He who began a good work in her was carrying it to completion (Philippians 1:6), and her flourishing had little to do with me and my best efforts.

If we want people to change, we can't just point out their short-comings and demand better behavior. We get to focus on growing in love *for* them and pray for change that is truly in the interest of their flourishing, not merely in line with our own agenda. Isn't that what we'd want for ourselves?

Through prayer, I surrendered my failed efforts to change Haley. I accepted that reforming her was not within my capacity. I released my plans and instead tried to align them with God's. Prayer renewed my ability to love her selflessly and support the work that God was doing in her life.

Paul wanted people to change too. He desperately wanted people to receive the gospel and to follow Jesus. When he wanted to see change, he leaned on prayer:

"We have not ceased to pray for you, asking that you may be filled with the knowledge of his will in all spiritual wisdom and understanding, so as to walk in a manner worthy of the Lord, fully pleasing to him: bearing fruit in every good work and increasing in the knowledge of God" (Colossians 1:9–10 ESV).

Paul was so committed to praying for the Colossians because he understood that the changing of hearts was God's work. Walking "in a manner worthy of the Lord," as Paul put it, was the fruit of knowing God, not the result of being bullied into submission by a well-meaning sister. God, it turns out, is the One cultivating the fruit—not me.

When we hope to see change in others, we jumpstart change by transforming our own hearts toward them. We do this through prayer, for their blessing and for their growth. Prayer corrected my beliefs about my own capacity and renewed my energy to support my sister. When I surrendered my efforts to control and change Haley, I found that my exhaustion around our relationship dissipated. And no surprise, I am a much better big sister. When I set my heart on her good, I surrendered my misguided efforts to fix her; I found peace in knowing God would do the work that only He is able to do.

The reality that "I am not enough" to fix someone else becomes freeing, not disheartening. Where our attempts to fix people leave us burned out, prayer imparts energy and frees us up to walk alongside them in love.

Let's start now.

Lord,
Thank You for how You are at work in the changing of hearts and minds, and that You want to use me in others' lives. I ask You for humility and for sincerity in my desire for others' good. Use me to draw in others, and correct me when I push others away. I am setting my eyes on Your redemptive power, surrendering my anxiety about my loved ones into Your hands.
Amen.

27

Too Much Information

Travel back in time with me to 2020. This was no one's favorite year. We experienced collective trauma on a global scale. Millions died, and millions more grew ill. We didn't know how dangerous the virus was, and we certainly didn't know how long we'd be in lockdown. We cancelled graduations and weddings. Kids attended school virtually for multiple years. I came *so* close to delivering my first baby all alone in a California hospital, surrounded by doctors in HAZMAT suits.

Seemingly overnight, the world was driven indoors and onto our devices. Along with everyone else, I was reading the news almost daily. I clicked on article after article, reading updates about the pandemic, reports of racial injustice and subsequent protests, details of the current political drama (of which there was no shortage), and articles about rising geopolitical tensions around the globe. Difficult news was made worse by a vitriolic social media climate, full of strong opinions that were light on information. It was harrowing, and yet I couldn't look away.

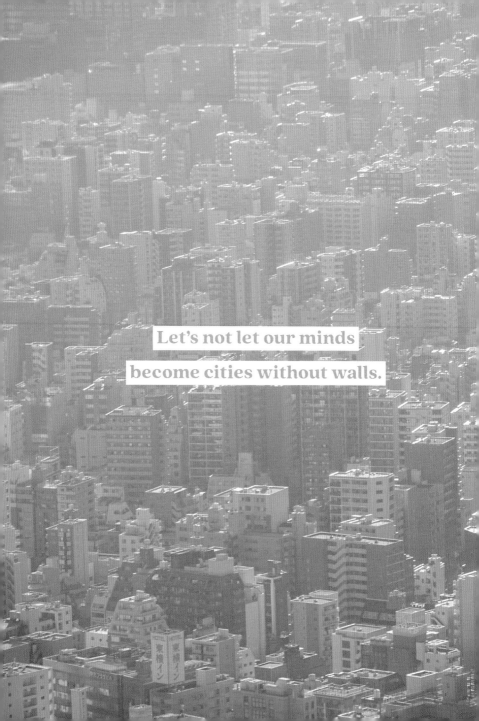

Let's not let our minds become cities without walls.

Suddenly, I knew a lot about everything—or so I felt—and my mind was rarely still. My anxiety about the state of the world skyrocketed, until one day, I didn't feel a thing. I'd scroll through stories of death and destruction, and yet I would feel nothing.

I wasn't a monster; I was just burned out.

Being informed wasn't the problem. Being constantly inundated with information from my TV and phone and tablet, on top of the emotional distress from being stuck in isolation—*that* was the problem. It still is.

I just checked my screentime stats, and at present, my daily average is just over seven hours. *Seven!* Of course, some of that time is from work, texting friends, and FaceTiming family members, but for much of it, I am just scrolling through social media feeds and news headlines. I often find myself tossed from a tragic news headline to an inflammatory meme to a college friend's pregnancy announcement, all in the span of five minutes. My poor brain is doing her best, but she can't possibly manage to process all the information *and* feel a full range of emotions. Our minds don't have the capacity for all this data, and our hearts can't keep up with our scrolling.

What are we to do? Being informed and aware enables us to meet the needs in the world; burying our heads in the sand isn't the answer. No, instead of swearing off information in all its forms, the solution lies in setting limits around our mindless consumption of content.

"Like a city breached, without walls, is one who lacks self-control" (Proverbs 25:28 NRSV).

Let's not allow our minds become cities without walls. When

it comes to doomscrolling and mindless media consumption, we need self-control to keep us safe and healthy. There is some nuance here because our individual boundaries will all look different. Your job is to be honest with yourself when media consumption is no longer helpful.

The good news is the Bible teaches that we have a tool at our disposal to help us with this discernment: "For God gave us a spirit not of fear but of power and love and self-control" (2 Timothy 1:7 ESV). The information at our fingertips is a gift, so long as we maintain that spirit of power and love and self-control. In the context of social media, employing a spirit of self-control can help us regain a sense of agency. We can set boundaries around how much time we spend online and where we source our news, using any extra time for self-reflection and prayer for how to steward the information we're taking in.

Your limitations are a gift, even if they don't always feel like it. It's okay to take a break. It's wise to go outside and stop dwelling on all that's wrong in the world. Yes, we should stay informed, but know it's okay to look away sometimes. Where you focus your attention matters, for what you do and for who you are. Find rest in your limits, and honor how God made you.

Lord,
Show me how to set healthy limits for
information. Grow me in self-control, and
give me the discernment to know when I've
reached my capacity. Help me live according
to the spirit of power and love and self-
control You have given me. Thank You that
I don't have to carry all of this alone.
Amen.

WE CAN'T

LET THE

OVERWHELM

WIN!

Stoplight

Recently, God made me really uncomfortable in the best way while reading Matthew 25:35–36, which says: "For I was hungry and you gave me something to eat, I was thirsty and you gave me something to drink, I was a stranger and you invited me in, I needed clothes and you clothed me, I was sick and you looked after me, I was in prison and you came to visit me" (NIV). I started thinking about who I was feeding, clothing, and visiting. The list was pretty short.

Driving around my city, I prayed, "God, who am I supposed to be feeding and clothing?"

At the stoplight, I looked up. There was a woman standing there on the corner, two kids beside her, with a sign asking for money to feed her kids. There was need. Right in front of me.

In a very awkward effort to just be obedient to Scripture, I rolled down my window. "Hey, I don't have cash, but is there anything you need from the store?" I said, gesturing to the grocery store down the block.

"Water, please," she said, which made sense in the one-hundred-degree summer heat. "And we don't have anywhere to sleep."

So I went to the store. I bought water bottles. I threw in some snacks for her kids. I added a gift card, hoping to help with future needs. I inquired with my church about local organizations that could help her get a hotel room for the night and hopefully more long-term assistance. I wrote down some phone numbers.

Then I went back, handed her the bag of groceries, and got their names. I asked if I could pray for them.

I don't deserve a lot of credit for this good deed because it wasn't that hard. It's surprisingly simple to respond to the needs in front of us. Ever since that encounter, I have been rolling down my window more. I may only have a protein bar to offer, but I want to make sure that I am acknowledging the humanity in front of me. At the very least, I want to know these individuals' names and how I can pray for them.

Later in Matthew 25, Jesus said, "Truly I tell you, whatever you did not do for one of the least of these, you did not do for me" (v. 45 NIV). As Christians, we are called to search for Jesus' face in the faces of people in need all around us. I worry that we have forgotten what it means to *see* someone who needs help and just help them. But when we do, we're ministering to folks who bear God's image.

In John 6, Jesus multiplied one willing little boy's bread and fishes to feed thousands. With that boy's small act of faith and obedience, Jesus did something miraculous. What if we adopted the same heart of this little boy, giving our resources freely?

The world is overwhelming, but we can't let the overwhelm win! We are inundated with information, aware of so many needs. I often feel paralyzed, unsure where to focus my attention, but then I realize I only have to look right outside my window. I bring what I have to the people right in front of me and entrust my loaves and fishes to Christ.

If you see a hungry person, help them get food. If you see someone outside in the cold without a coat, can you offer one from your closet to help them get warm? If you see someone who feels like "the other"—whether due to racial, economic, or social reasons—reach out in an act of hospitality *in that moment*. And if you see someone struggling, say, "Hey, I know you're having a hard time. Knowing Jesus changed everything for me, so I am here if you want to talk."

God has equipped us for this, friends! The Holy Spirit is with us! When we jump into God's work in the world, our own faith grows because we get to see Him working. God has chosen to use us in small ways that He, in His power and limitless strength and wisdom, multiplies into world change.

Jesus,
I want to make a difference in the world,
and I want to follow You well. Open my eyes
to the need around me as I move through my
day. Give me the boldness to believe that You
have equipped me to engage with that need,
and to love You as I serve others. You can
multiply whatever I bring to You in faith.
Amen.

Super Fast

My toddler, Judah, doesn't stop moving. Ever. He kicked constantly in the womb. He walked at ten months old. He climbs to the top of thirty-foot play structures with zero hesitation. The other day, he jumped off a fifteen-foot platform at a trampoline park, completely unassisted. He is *two*.

So of course he's in love with the word "super." One day we were walking in the park, and he looked up at me, excited. "Mama, Judah go *super* fast!" He then proceeded to run as fast as his little legs could go—an enthusiastic, uncoordinated little power walk. In his mind he is an Olympic sprinter, but to me he just looks like an awkward little penguin, waddling as fast as he can.

When I watch him, I can't help but wonder if this is what I look like to God when I try to hustle my way into success and happiness. I feel pressured to have a well-formed career path, a profitable side hustle, a thriving social life, an aesthetic home, healthy spiritual habits, a regular fitness regimen, and a marriage that weathers no rough patches. I make to-do lists I can never finish, but I load up on coffee and try my hardest. *I can survive on five hours of sleep*, I tell myself.

This is my *super*-fast life.

To God, who has already determined my path, my big plans and power moves are the equivalent of an adorably awkward toddler.

What are we even hustling toward? Happiness? One study found that up to 70 percent of high-level executives are considering leaving their high-powered jobs in favor of ones that are easier on their mental well-being (Dennison 2022). It seems the people who achieved the goals and the promotions are just as burned out as the rest of us.

We are working and working to produce fulfillment in our lives. Our hustle isn't working, but we keep going anyway. So let me disrupt this never-ending cycle for you today: God didn't design you to work yourself into fulfillment; God designed you to find fulfillment resting in Him.

The American Dream tells us, "Work hard and you can have it all"; the gospel says, "Christ is your all, and His grace is a free gift." The rampant consumerism around us wants us to believe that more money and more stuff is proof of success, and by extension, it is a sign of God's favor.

Hear Jesus' words to the hustlers and the strivers and the hard workers in Matthew 11: "Come to me, all you who are weary and burdened, and I will give you rest. Take my yoke upon you and learn from me, for I am gentle and humble in heart, and you will find rest for your souls. For my yoke is easy and my burden is light" (vv. 28–31 NIV).

You cannot
work your way
to real rest.

Jesus was speaking to working-class people who woke up day after day to do back-breaking physical labor. Can you imagine trying to make sense of these words after a day in the fields? Here's this man, claiming that He can relieve you of endless work, claiming that He's going to give you an easier burden to carry?

Jesus was trying to teach us something we still haven't learned, even centuries later: When we know true rest, our labor becomes meaningful. When our identity is tied to Christ and not our profession, we can live lives of peace and fulfillment, a privilege given *to* us and unable to be earned *by* us.

What does that look like? It's choosing to walk slowly and linger on beauty because often that beauty is where God reveals Himself. It means relishing God's kind gifts, sometimes even instead of working.

So long as we are trying to earn fulfillment through hustling, we will find ourselves burned out and frustrated. Today, as you engage in your work, don't forget to take your eyes off the grind sometimes. Embrace the liberating reality that, in your own strength, you cannot ever work your way to real rest. Look to Jesus and believe that the easy yoke will bring the fulfillment you've been after all along.

Lord,
Free me from the pressure to produce
and achieve. The world around me continues
to yell that if I can only work a little harder
and a little later, I will finally have a life I
love. I know in my heart this cannot be true,
that You alone are the way to find rest and
fulfillment. I am taking my eyes off hustle
culture, and I am giving You that heavy yoke.
Amen.

Abiding is the opposite of hustling.

Wait to Grow

Plant girlies, please tell me how you keep those things alive. Every plant I have ever owned has lived a short, beautiful beginning that culminated in a slow, languishing end. In my head, I am one of you—a plant mom. In real life, I am a plant killer.

I am also the mother to two humans who seem to be surviving just fine, so riddle me that. When it comes to plants, though, I get stressed about how to care for them. I am always watering them too little or far too much. I put them in the wrong kind of pot. I leave the ones that need shade in the direct sunlight. Inevitably, after a few weeks, I see my once-promising plant starting to wilt. I know death is imminent.

My sister, on the other hand, has the entire rainforest living in her home. The ficuses are flourishing. The succulents are succeeding. The pothos is prospering.

From my experience killing numerous plants, I have learned one important principle: the most meaningful growth requires proper nourishment and rest. The same is true of our spiritual lives. In order to grow, God tells us we need to nourish ourselves and rest in His presence:

"Abide in me, and I in you. As the branch cannot bear fruit by itself, unless it abides in the vine, neither can you, unless you abide in me. I am the vine; you are the branches. Whoever abides in me and I in him, he it is that bears much fruit, for apart from me you can do nothing. If anyone does not abide in me he is thrown away like a branch and withers; and the branches are gathered, thrown into the fire, and burned" (John 15:4–6 ESV).

What does it mean to "abide"? The simplest definition is "to dwell"—to remain, to stay. In plant terms, like those Jesus chooses in John 15, to abide is to remain connected to our Source. We pretend that we are in control of our spiritual growth, but really, the only piece we control is how much we surrender to God amid the unknowns.

Abiding is the diametric opposite of hustling.

When you abide in God's presence, strengthening your relationship with Him through time in prayer and absorbing Scripture, you will encounter a new kind of power. Jesus promises to sustain you for a meaningful life full of fruit and purpose. Being connected to God means a constant source of supernatural power and resilience.

As you abide, you may discover you need to prune the things that compromise your focus and fidelity—to kill the weeds, if you will. Your achievements, titles, awards, or anything else that distracts you from resting in God's presence and following His teachings? They must go. Only then can the Gardener do His true work in you.

He can use you to revive the heart of your neighbor. He can use you to bring life back into a community that might be struggling. He can use you in any number of amazing ways to reinvigorate the broken world we live in through your specific gifts and passions.

God's power is always available, so long as you can remain

connected to the Source of your life—Jesus Christ. This doesn't mean life will be easy or that you'll never feel tired again. Your responsibilities may still be demanding, but God promises to give you strength. You will still experience pain, but your Source of life will always remain safe and secure. Your struggles may still push you to your limit, but so long as you abide in Him, you can trust that your future is secure.

Seek to abide; set your eyes on God. Stay close, stay connected. I promise you, anxious though your heart may be, God will bring about the results your heart desires when you surrender your hustle into His hand.

TODAY'S READING: JOHN 15:1–17
FOR ADDITIONAL STUDY: ROMANS 8:5–11

Father,
I want to flourish and grow. I want You to be the Gardener. The future You have ordained is the future I want; the fruit You can bring about is the fruit I want to bear. Help me set my eyes on You and Your work as I seek to remain connected to You. I trust You will bring the growth if I stay connected.
Amen.

PART 4

Scarcity + Abundance

There never seems to be enough.

Not enough money. Not enough energy. Certainly not enough time. It feels like the opportunities we desire go to someone else who is smarter or more qualified or just *better*.

Maybe it feels like all the "good" dating prospects are already taken. Or maybe you feel like you'll never catch up in your career.

I have often found myself spiraling around the belief that I do not have enough—not enough stuff, not enough talent, not enough charisma—you name it, I want it.

Often we put our attention on what we don't have and approach our days with an unspoken fear that we serve a God who withholds. We sometimes subconsciously believe that He's stingy, greedy, or waiting for us to be perfect before He will give us what our hearts desire.

Over the next ten days, we are going to explore the anxiety of this perpetual mindset of scarcity and, prayerfully, we will replace it with a vision of the abundance God provides. Let's retrain our focus away from the things we wrongly *think* will bring us contentment and instead set our gaze on *El Shaddai*—the God of All Sufficiency, the God of more than enough.

What if you really believed that He would provide for *you*, lovingly aware of every need that you have? How would that change your life?

Let's set our eyes on His abundance and find out.

For in Christ all the fullness of the Deity lives in bodily form, and in Christ you have been brought to fullness.

Colossians 2:9–10 NIV

Trust in the LORD and do good;
 dwell in the land and enjoy safe pasture.
Take delight in the LORD,
 and he will give you the desires of your heart.

Psalm 37:3–4 NIV

Remember this: Whoever sows sparingly will also reap sparingly, and whoever sows generously will also reap generously. Each of you should give what you have decided in your heart to give, not reluctantly or under compulsion, for God loves a cheerful giver. And God is able to bless you abundantly, so that in all things at all times, having all that you need, you will abound in every good work.

2 Corinthians 9:6–8 NIV

Fleeting Fulfillment

For one surreal moment, I felt contentment.
I had been waiting and searching and hoping, and I had achieved
it. I wasn't looking around for new solutions anymore; no, I had
found the answer to my problems. Life had changed. I stared at my
husband, disbelief in my eyes.

"You . . . bought me the Airwrap?"

I could have cried. We couldn't afford this splurge, but my
husband knew I had been struggling to feel cute after giving birth.
I had showed him videos proving that this product was going to
change my life. I tried to find used ones to purchase secondhand.

My parents were both in the advertising industry, and I have a
natural skepticism toward marketing. But the Dyson Airwrap . . .
oh, they got me. I was convinced that my hair would never know
frizz again. I would finally have the volume I had always wanted.
This product—well outside my normal budget for hair care—
would alter the course of my future.

How do I feel a year later? Look, it's a great product. I like it a lot. But the Airwrap did not change my DNA. My hair is still my hair.

I think now, maybe more than ever, we're tempted to seek fulfillment and life change through accumulating stuff—whether makeup or memberships or clothes or technology. Nearly every influencer ad I see starts with some variation of "This product is life-changing." And even though I know better, part of me believes it. *Add to cart.*

The marketing industry knows that appealing to our fears of not having or being enough is a great way to pique our interest. They then make us believe that maybe there is hope for us in the form of their product!

We try to fix our feelings of deficiency by accumulating *things*, but true abundance and having lots of stuff are not the same thing. Living from abundance means proclaiming, "I have enough," even when the ads and the influencers are getting under your skin.

To move from a materialism and scarcity mindset to contentment and abundance will require us to reframe what provision really means. Paul reminds us that, "We brought nothing into the world, and we can take nothing out of it. But if we have food and clothing, we will be content with that" (1 Timothy 6:7–8 NIV). It is very easy in Western consumer culture for our little "wants" to morph into perceived "needs."

Indeed, there is something sacred about needing. Explore your needs. Are they actually "needs," or are they "wants"? Both are okay, but we are wise to be clearheaded about which is which so that we do not become entangled in a culture of consumerism.

That said, God can fulfill both your "needs" and your "wants." Digging into your desires can be a good and beautiful thing. Let your wants and needs drive you closer to God in prayer and deeper into reliance on Him.

If your treasure is found in God, your heart will be content in His abundance (Matthew 6:21). If your treasure is found in material things, you will feel deficient and anxious.

Until your heart believes this, consider setting some parameters around social media and shopping platforms that make it so easy to feed your hunger for *more*. New stuff will give you a short-lived high but will ultimately leave you wondering where all your money went and antsy about how you'll afford all the other unnecessary "essentials" you don't really need. This desire for more keeps you locked in a cycle of scarcity.

Allow me to de-influence you: if you didn't like your hair before the Dyson Airwrap, you probably won't like it after you get one. "Must-have" activewear will not suddenly transform your negative thoughts about your body. Your heart will still be hungry, even if you have the financial ability to buy items from every single Amazon Storefront you stumble across.

No amount of money—and nothing you could buy—will bring you sustained contentment. Ask God to retrain your eyes to discern true needs, and pray that He would give you a heart of gratitude for the many things He has already provided.

Dear Lord,
I see how You have provided for me
and blessed me beyond what I deserve. I
still find myself weighed down by desires
for more than I need. Help me to stop
focusing on what I don't have. Help me shift
my gaze away from all the things I lack to
find abundance right in front of me.
Amen.

Unclenching Our Fists

I wanted to cry as I slapped a shipping label on a box containing one of my favorite dresses. I had sold it on a popular resale app, and it was time to send it to its new owner. Part of me was sad, but a bigger part of me felt free.

After hearing a convicting sermon about consumerism, the Lord laid an idea on my heart: What if I listed every *single* thing in my closet on this resale app for ninety days? What if I gave the money I made selling my clothing to people in need?

I would simplify my closet. I would break my attachment to my stuff. I would do tangible things to care for people in my community. Check, check, and check.

Of course, this project didn't always feel good. I had invested a lot of money into my closet, and to watch it dwindle was tough. As you can imagine, the items that sold first were usually the most current and in-demand brand names, which of course were the things I liked most. I ached when I got each notification of a new sale.

Scarcity proved itself a liar.

As much as it hurt, I desperately wanted my life to be aligned with God's priorities, to live into the abundant reality of God's provision of kingdom terms and not on the terms of our never-enough economy. Every time I got rid of another piece of clothing, I noticed how I felt a little freer. Each time I shipped off another item, I was reminded that I had plenty of clothes left in my closet, and that my true identity had nothing to do with my clothes.

With the money I made, I purchased gift cards that I kept in my purse for people needing money or food. Did I solve poverty? Obviously not. But for me, this was a spiritual discipline that showed how God could use me when I loosened my clenched fists from my possessions. My clothes—even my favorite ones—were so temporary in their value to me. When I converted those clothes into resources to serve others, I felt like God was using me for something *real*. In that teeny-tiny act of surrender, God did so much to shift my gaze to the real abundance found in giving away.

While I did sell most of my favorite items, I never felt like my closet was deficient. In fact, when I stopped looking to new clothes for that quick, easy hit of dopamine, I found myself open to all the ways God orchestrated new and unique blessings in my life. Whether it was a beautiful sunset or a coffee with a friend, I realized that God has absolutely no problem bringing beauty into my life. Scarcity proved itself a liar, and God proved Himself faithful.

I couldn't have predicted the divine provision and freedom I'd experience when I let go of my possessions. God wired us for abundance—for the peace that comes with knowing "there is enough" and the freedom that comes when we trust Him to meet our needs. We forget that peace and freedom can only be found in Him, not in things we collect.

As Jesus told the crowd in Luke 12:15, "Watch out! Be on your guard against all kinds of greed; life does not consist in an abundance of possessions" (NIV). You will not find the abundance you seek in *stuff*. In fact, you will only encounter abundance in your life when you loosen your grip and learn to give.

Don't believe me? Read Proverbs 11:24–25: "There is one who scatters, and yet increases all the more, and there is one who withholds what is justly due, and yet it results only in poverty. A generous person will be prosperous, and one who gives others plenty of water will himself be given plenty" (NASB).

Any need you're trying to buy the solution for right now? God is already committed to meeting it! God wants you to enjoy your life, friend. Trust Him for this!

If we waste our time on the counterfeit abundance of collecting stuff, we will miss the true abundance found in giving. Only when we hold our possessions loosely will we notice God providing unexpectedly and abundantly in ways that equip us to see and respond to the material needs of others.

Lord,
I want to make space in my life to see
You lovingly meeting my needs. Help me
release my grip on material things to take
hold of Your provision and priorities. Help
me set my eyes on all the ways You are loving
me and drawing me into abundance.
Amen.

Wish You Were Her

Let's talk about envy. I'd really prefer not to, if I'm being honest. I can remember on multiple occasions explaining to people that, "I'm not a jealous person!" because I have rarely experienced the pang of frustration or sadness that comes when I see someone else get something good. If I don't resent others when they have good things, I must not have a problem.

Or so I thought. I have been deeply unhappy with myself at times, wishing to be more like others. For example, I don't think I'm a natural beauty; I have longed to wake up gorgeous like my friend Destiny. I have never felt like people gravitate to me; there are times I would have given anything for the charming personality of my friend Sara. My friend Rachel laughs so easily—that girl is always lighthearted, always having fun. Why can't I make people laugh like *her*? Why can't I have better posture like *her*? Why can't I be creative like *her*?

It's not that I don't think I have good qualities; it's that others

YOU WERE NOT MADE
TO SPEND YOUR
DAYS WISHING
FOR THE GIFTS OF
ANOTHER.

always seem to shine brighter. My envy flew under the radar because, unlike our classic ideas of jealousy, I didn't harbor bitterness toward other people. Instead, my bitterness and my discontent were directed at how *God* chose to make me. I have often lived from that place of scarcity, believing if God made me just a little more pretty, smart, hardworking, athletic, kind, or funny, then my life would be better.

This is what happens when a mentality of scarcity creeps into how we see ourselves. We fixate on how we are not enough and how others seem to have more. We dismiss the good God has created in us and question why He created others so much "better."

You cannot be anyone except who God made you to be. Every day you spend trying to be more like someone else is a day you miss living in the beauty God implanted in *you*. God loves each of us uniquely, and every time we devalue ourselves, we are disrespecting Him and the plan He has ordained for our lives.

In Isaiah 45, God convicted Israel of their doubt that He could accomplish His purposes through them, the humans He created. The prophet Isaiah wrote, "Woe to those who quarrel with their Maker. . . . Does the clay say to the potter, 'What are you making?' Does your work say, 'The potter has no hands'?" (Isaiah 45:9 NIV).

It would be ridiculous to think that a pot could critique the potter; the potter is the one who thought up the design and the purpose and chose the materials. When the pot starts wishing it had a spout here or a handle there, the pot is wishing away the purpose it was designed for. This pot could spend its whole life trying to be a pitcher or a vase or a mug, but the pot would always feel defective. When it surrenders to the design of the potter, the pot will find abundance in the role and purpose it was created for.

I know I'm being *really* subtle with the metaphor here, but if you've missed it: *you* are the pot. He is the Potter. If you want to find joy and experience the abundance of how God created you individually, you will have to learn how to admire qualities in others without coveting them as your own.

I am certain of this: you were not made to spend your days wishing for the gifts of another. God made you, *you*! With *your* qualities and *your* gifts and, yes, even your struggles—for good and beautiful things. I am begging you not to waste the beauty of who you are by believing God did a better job on someone else.

TODAY'S READING: ISAIAH 45:9–12

FOR ADDITIONAL STUDY: PSALM 139:13–18

God,
I struggle to see my value and purpose. I don't always believe that You made me good. I wish I had what she has—I want the gifts and the blessings I see You providing to others. I am tired of looking at others with envy in my heart. Renew my perspective; set my eyes on the good You designed in and for me.
Amen.

You Have Everything You Need

My husband sometimes wishes he had gone to a different school for his master's degree. It's not that he hated his experience; in fact, he loved the church he attended, and his roommate from that time is still one of his favorite people. But in his early twenties, just out of college and a thousand miles from home, he had difficulty figuring out his finances, beliefs, and personal goals. His experience in seminary challenged his personal beliefs—and, let's face it, was also pretty expensive (which I did not realize until after we got married and combined bank accounts . . . but now I can confirm with an unfortunate level of confidence).

Who among us doesn't have regrets?

Have you ever felt a pang of regret as you looked back at a big life choice, feeling the sting of "what if"? Well, here's the thing: these regrets are just another version of scarcity making its way into your heart and controlling how you experience joy. You may believe that you made one wrong choice along the way and that you messed up God's plan. You believe you only had a tiny handful of chances to be something great, and you blew it. There's just that *one* path that God mapped out for you, and after you messed up, God moved on to someone who has better navigation skills.

Let me assure you: God wasn't surprised by your choice then, and He will have no problem redeeming that choice now. God can take any set of circumstances and use them for your good and His glory.

For example, my husband, Tanner, may have struggled attending a seminary of different theological leanings from his own. He was frequently exhausted having to answer questions and settle debates. But now, Tanner is *the guy* you want on your team if you're navigating a fraught theological topic. Because of his seminary experience, he is well-versed in all sides of big theological debates. More importantly, he's humble and exceedingly charitable to those who disagree with him. In seminary Tanner realized that most of us are just doing our best. His educational background has been a huge asset in his current ministry role.

Look, I know it's hard to see the big picture on a plain-old Tuesday and, honestly, we may never get a detailed explanation of how God works everything together for our good. But He's been doing this work for all eternity, and the Bible presents us with God's good track record. We can trust Him to bring about His purposes in and through us. And we can trust that those purposes will be far more beautiful and worthwhile than spending our lives consumed with regret and comparison.

Cling to this truth: "His divine power has given us *everything we need* for a godly life through our knowledge of him who called us by his own glory and goodness. Through these he has given us his very great and precious promises, so that through them you may participate in the divine nature, having escaped the corruption in the world caused by evil desires" (2 Peter 1:3–4 NIV, emphasis added).

God has given you everything you need for a godly life, regardless of your regrets and "what-ifs." This promise isn't conditional. The Bible doesn't say, "As long as you are perfect and never depart from God's plan for your life." No! From the moment you invite God's power into your circumstances through prayer and submission to His teaching, you will see His power to orchestrate opportunity, lead you to the next step, and cultivate contentment in your heart. You can't miss it.

We can waste time longing for our circumstances and the choices of our past to be different, or we can allow God to use our gifts to their fullest and to help us shine in the gifts He has ordained for us. We can dwell in regret—that is, scarcity—or we can embrace God's abundant power for today. Rest in the knowledge that God will offer you more chances than you'll ever need to fulfill His purpose for your life. Surrender—or re-surrender for the tenth (or hundredth) time—your circumstances, and see what He can do.

Lord,
You have ordained plans for me as a unique
individual. I am trusting that all of this will
make sense one day, and that for now, all I can
do is surrender to Your work. Help me to get
excited about what You are doing in my life
so I can be free from comparison and envy. I
am setting my eyes on Your plans for me.
Amen.

On Friend Group Shows

Let me take you on a journey to the early twenty-first century, when teen television was at its prime. In the pre-streaming days, season premieres were events you marked on your calendar. We had to wait an entire week in between episodes, and it was *torture*.

My favorite shows were "friend group" shows, by which I mean shows about a group of friends (always beautiful, generally wealthy, rarely supervised) who get into trouble, kiss each others' significant others, and party at the one extra-rich friend's vacation house. *Gossip Girl, One Tree Hill, The OC*—these were my shows. The drama was utterly unhinged, but the friends always came back together in the end.

Sign me up, thirteen-year-old me thought.

I can trace my desire to have a friend group to these series. I have always wanted a community who knows me and accepts me, go-to cohorts for vacations, double dates, and now, multi-family barbecues on holidays.

I think we all want to feel deeply known. We want to know where we fit and who we can trust. Unfortunately, acquiring those things feels hard. It doesn't help that TV, and now social media, offer a romanticized vision of how cool your life would be if you had such a group. It seems like everyone else has one!

And yet, we are lonelier than ever. As of 2023, the US Surgeon General named loneliness an epidemic with significant physical health complications. Based on the numbers, loneliness is just as deadly as smoking up to fifteen cigarettes per day (HHS 2023). How is it possible that we could be more connected than ever and yet are simultaneously dying from the effects of emotional isolation?

What I fear is the belief that the only friendships worth having are marked by constant entertainment. We have been fed unrealistic standards. It seems that if we don't have beautiful or exciting friendships that we can post about, then why bother? Friendship has become more about what others do for us than it is about the richness of knowing another human being. Who cares if we have friends if we can't show off what we do together? Doesn't it seem that way? So we pre-judge people and end up lonely.

Sounds like scarcity to me. "I don't have any friends!" we lament. "There's no one I connect with at my school/church/etc." Actually, we are frequently surrounded by people, many of whom we know little about. Is it possible that we are looking for friends with the wrong criteria in mind? Judging their worth before knowing it?

Community and friendship are good desires that God wired into the human heart (Genesis 2:18). God wants to give them to you.

"Which of you, if your son asks for bread, will give him a stone? Or if he asks for a fish, will give him a snake? If you, then, though you are evil, know how to give good gifts to your children, how much more will your Father in heaven give good gifts to those who ask him!" (Matthew 7:9–11 NIV).

Is it possible that God has answered our prayers, and that we're missing it? That we are willing to be lonely instead of giving different kinds of friends a try?

When I was in my early twenties, I stumbled into friendship with a few moms in their forties and fifties. At first, I didn't think of them as friends. They weren't my age. We had totally different schedules, interests, and views. But my "mom friends" (as I endearingly refer to them) came through for me when I was struggling with motherhood. When I was too anxious to be home alone with my new baby, they would bring me dinner, rock Judah, clean my kitchen, and pray over me. Intergenerational friendships are amazing.

Maybe you are lacking community. But what if, for the sake of experiment, you opened your heart to friendships with people you normally wouldn't?

Try going out of your way to check in with your elderly neighbor. Chat just a little bit longer with the overbearing pastor's wife (hi, it's me!). Yes, it may feel weird, but you might be shocked at how many would-be friends God has already placed around you. Fighting loneliness (and with it, and our scarcity mindset around community) might not have to be so hard.

Dear Lord,
I pray that You would free me from loneliness
by surrounding me with abundant community.
Help me open my heart to the people You place
around me. Expand my vision of friendship. Take
my eyes off my limited idea of community, and set
my eyes on the abundance You have provided.
Amen.

Rejecting Scarcity

If you've met my mother, you know she's a host. When people are coming to her home, she will clean every single inch of it on the off chance that her guest requests a tour. She'll craft the right playlist and arrange fresh flowers. She spares no expense on the food selection for the evening. If you ever receive an invite to the residence of Amy Pierson, you can expect the *good* plates and a special dessert. I learned from the best, and so did she—my grandmother was a legend for her hospitality.

I'll be honest—growing up, I didn't understand why my mom made such a big deal about hosting guests. Sometimes, it felt like a lot of work for what seemed to be minimal payoff. Personally, I would have preferred a reservation at a restaurant and a hard stop after ninety minutes of chatting.

Now, I get it. We put effort into hosting because it demonstrates honor. We invite people in as a tangible picture of openness and warmth. Hospitality lays the groundwork for relationship, and therefore, community. For me, opening up my home has proven uncomfortably vulnerable too. I rarely have time to clean everything the way I'd like, and honestly, sometimes a huge, fancy spread of food isn't in our budget. When you walk through my door, you walk right past the curated facade I'd prefer to project.

In these ways and many more, hospitality is a refusal to live from a place of scarcity. The extra time, energy, and money we spend may feel like they're in short supply on a given day; choosing to host and serve others anyway—that's an act of defiance to every "not-enough" feeling. Hospitality says, "Yes, there is enough. There's always enough." We see firsthand how choosing abundance begets more abundance; giving of ourselves paves the way for laughter, memories, and relationship. In giving of ourselves, we encounter blessing (Acts 20:35).

Hospitality is the antidote to loneliness plaguing our world. God is calling us, His people, to make the first move. In an act of radical hospitality, Jesus washed the feet of His disciples, and then commanded them to go and do likewise (John 13:12–15). So we actively seek out others and invite them into an environment of warmth and welcome, regardless of setting.

Take it from Jesus: "When you give a luncheon or dinner, do not invite your friends, your brothers or sisters, your relatives, or your rich neighbors; if you do, they may invite you back and so you will be repaid. But when you give a banquet, invite the poor, the crippled, the lame, the blind, and you will be blessed. Although they cannot repay you, you will be repaid at the resurrection of the righteous" (Luke 14:12–14 NIV).

Hospitality, then, is about leaving our comfort zones to extend

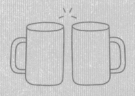

HOSPITALITY IS THE
ANTIDOTE TO LONELINESS.

welcome to people we might otherwise ignore. It requires us to stop evaluating people based on what they can offer us or how they fit into our romanticized vision of community. It requires us to let God surprise us with what He can do with our yes.

I can almost hear the introverts groaning. Trust me, even though we host people at least once a week, I (*an extrovert!*) still find myself dragging my feet when I think about the preparation and the small talk and the cleanup. Hospitality isn't easy; few things worth doing are. But remember: abundance begets abundance. When you engage in sacrificial hospitality—the kind that seeks out friendship in unexpected places—I promise you, you'll find *your* life enriched as well. After all, "Whoever brings blessing will be enriched, and one who waters will himself be watered" (Proverbs 11:25 ESV).

Trust that God can and will show up when you say yes to radical hospitality. Little by little, you'll watch community form and relationships grow. Bit by bit, the loneliness will cease to loom so large.

Dear God,
Today, I reject the scarcity mindset that says
I don't have the space or time to open my heart
or home. Show me who I can welcome; lead me
to the stranger who You would have me invite.
Train my heart in true hospitality, and allow me
to experience the abundance on the other side.
Amen.

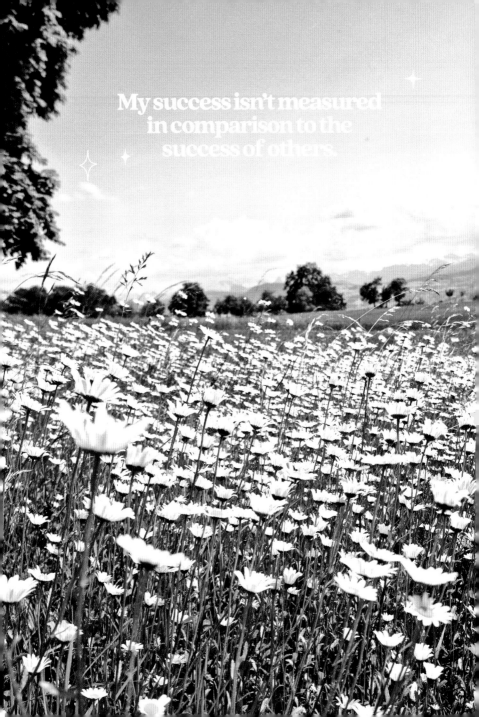

My success isn't measured
in comparison to the
success of others.

Running Behind

I recently opened my eighth-grade journal and found a long list of goals. As an achievement-oriented firstborn, I experienced no shortage of affirmation, and I had the preposterous confidence to match. "You can do anything you set your mind to!" my parents and teachers all said, and twelve-year-old me replied, "Watch me."

(A Selection of) Whitney's Goals:

#1: Be a camp counselor. (I actually achieved this. I will pause for your applause.)

#2: Be class valedictorian. (My GPA was okay, but this did not happen.)

#3: Start a charity. (I mean, this could still happen?)

#4: Be on the *Forbes* "30 Under 30" list.

That *Forbes* one tells you everything you need to know. Why was an eighth grader even reading *Forbes*? (*Forbes* is a business magazine, and every year they publish a "30 Under 30" list, which they say is "the definitive list of young people changing the world.") I was sure, given all the potential everyone was telling me I had, I would be able to make that list.

Well, guess who just turned thirty and—breaking news—never got that shout-out from *Forbes*! You may be shocked to hear this, but I have not accomplished many of my middle school goals. Sometimes it stings to realize that my life might come as a letdown to young, starry-eyed me. The truth is that, even though I have different goals, I still want to be extraordinary. And I feel like I am so far behind.

I have friends from college who are now completing PhDs. At one point, I thought I might be right there with them. I have friends with high-powered careers and the salaries to match. They're purchasing luxury cars and buying second homes, while my husband and I have to keep a pretty tight watch on our budget. Some days, I am not even sure what career path I am on, if I'm being honest.

All of it makes me feel like I am not keeping up. I look at others' success, and I feel like I should be so much further ahead. I am learning the hard way that the comparison game of fixing our eyes on others' success as a metric for our own is a form of scarcity. Comparison leaves us unable to enjoy the abundance of the individualized path God has paved for us. By measuring our lives in relation to others, we deny God's authority over our circumstances.

Second Corinthians 10:12–13 has been a balm to my soul: "We do not dare to classify or compare ourselves with some who commend themselves. When they measure themselves by themselves and compare themselves with themselves, they are not wise. We, however, will not boast beyond proper limits, but will confine our boasting to the sphere of service God himself has assigned to us, a sphere that also includes you" (NIV).

Paul wrote these words to the Corinthian church because, apparently, people were saying that he talked a big game in his letters but didn't deliver in person. He sounded assertive in writing but seemed humble in person. Paul, in response, explained that God had assigned him a specific area of service and that comparing himself to others was a waste of time. He refused to commend himself because he had nothing to prove.

Paul knew what I struggle to remember: I will never feel successful so long as I am comparing my accomplishments to others. Why? Because God hasn't called me to others' accomplishments. My success isn't measured in comparison to the success of others; my success is measured by how faithful I have been with what God has put in my "sphere of service."

Let me ask you a question I often ask myself: If God wants you to get that opportunity (or promotion, platform, paycheck, degree, etc.), don't you think He can make that happen? He is the God of the universe; doesn't it seem like He could elevate you at this very moment, should it align with His will? If you believe that He loves you (which I do), then what possible explanation is there for the fact that you are not further along?

Maybe it's because God wants you *exactly* where you are. Stop looking at others' success when God is trying to bless the space you're already standing in.

Lord,
Sometimes I get in my head and feel
inadequate compared to others. I feel behind—
like I missed something and can't catch up. I
am so exhausted from constantly measuring
myself against other people, with my eyes
set on them instead of on You. Help me trust
that You have me where I am for a purpose.
Amen.

No Shortcuts

I once was a renowned cross-country runner. My high school cross-country team was *huge*—about two hundred kids. Because the team was massive, the coaches mapped out a route and expected everyone to follow the person in front of them. The routes weaved through our nearby neighborhoods. So on any given route, someone knew a shortcut.

One day, all my effortlessly athletic fifteen-year-old guy friends took off toward a shortcut, and I did my best to keep up. I was not an effortlessly athletic fifteen-year-old boy, so I fell behind. Before I knew it, I was lost.

I didn't know the shortcut. I had no clue where I was supposed to go. We didn't carry our phones on these runs, so I tried to locate natural landmarks. At one point, I believe I attempted to track the movement of the sun, which is *news flash* not something I knew how to do. When I finally found my way back to the trail, I popped out from the "shortcut" and looked right up at my cross-country coach. He was *not* happy.

The punishment for cheating the course was sprinting laps

in front of the whole team, either four laps—a mile at a dead sprint—or a sixty-second quarter-mile. I ended up running three laps in a dead sprint. I nearly perished.

I also learned a pretty crucial life lesson: when my focus is on keeping up with others instead of on my course, I will likely end up lost.

God has an individual plan for each of us as specific as our DNA, and all that He requires is our "yes." God isn't looking around, worried that everyone else is faster:

"Therefore . . . let us run with perseverance the race marked out for us, fixing our eyes on Jesus, the pioneer and perfecter of faith. For the joy set before him he endured the cross, scorning its shame, and sat down at the right hand of the throne of God. Consider him who endured such opposition from sinners, so that you will not grow weary and lose heart" (Hebrews 12:1–3 NIV).

God has a course marked for you. If you keep your eyes on Christ, you might slow down, but you won't get lost. So don't lose heart. Christ pioneered your faith, and He is committed to perfecting it too. He knows what it's like to be hungry, rejected, adored, loved. He's run this human race. Jesus ran the course marked for Him—death on the cross—so that He could coach you as you run yours.

Turns out, I am a terrible long-distance runner and a mediocre sprinter, but I am a pretty decent mid-distance runner. When I stopped trying to keep up at any cost and focused on the path in front of me, I started to enjoy running. I accepted that sometimes I would be running alone, and I might have to work hard at it. When I showed up and submitted to the process, I figured out I can run a pretty fast mile. I found my own form of fulfillment and success when I focused on my own race.

You can't run well while you're constantly trying to take the routes meant for other people. Looking to your left and right for guidance will throw off your center of gravity and mess with your momentum. You must learn to run with your head steady and your eyes fixed on your goal. Comparing your place in the course to that of another runner will only slow you down.

Jesus has abundant joy set before you, friend. He wants you to flourish, so you can trust Him to guide your race. You might feel like you're in last place, but you might be at the right place and right time for a significant breakthrough.

When you feel anxious that you're moving too slow or like you've missed God's call for your life—when the lies of scarcity ring in your ears—I want you to remember you cannot run behind on His racecourse. So today, set your eyes on the Author and Perfecter, and put the next foot in front of the other.

Lord,
Help my heart believe that You have mapped my course. Help my heart look to You for assurance when I feel fear or doubt about my purpose. You can be trusted with my life, my calling, my career, and my plans. I am setting my eyes on Your sovereignty instead of my scarcity.
Amen.

Scarcity to Despair

Scarcity mentality is damaging, but never more so than when it creeps into how we see ourselves. When we find our inner dialogue shifting from *I will never have enough* to *I will never be enough*, despair is often close behind.

I've been there, and I will never forget it.

"I will do whatever it takes to be thin," I whispered. I was convinced to my core that I was deficient and, thus, unlovable.

I had "failed" in my obsessive diet plan and taken a bite of ice cream. That bite turned into a whole container. Later that night, my arms were wrapped around a toilet for the very first time. I had reached the point of despair, constantly focused on all the ways I didn't measure up. My eating disorder didn't begin that night. No, it had been months of dieting and obsessing over exercise in the making, but that was the night I surrendered to it. I just felt hopeless.

The eating disorder compelled me to spend my days looking at my perceived flaws. When we fixate on the scarcity, we will end up in a place of despair. These feelings of despair are on the rise across our culture (Graham). A recent study reports that over 44 percent of students deal with persistent feelings of hopelessness (CDC 2022). I was certainly part of that statistic. So I have to ask: Are you, the one sitting there holding this book, feeling this way too?

If you are, know this: we are not alone, and this hopelessness phenomenon isn't new. Paul had been there too: "For I have the desire to do what is good, but I cannot carry it out. . . . What a wretched man I am! Who will rescue me from this body that is subject to death?" (Romans 7:18, 24 NIV). He, too, found himself consumed with scarcity, lamenting that he was not enough to overcome sin and do good on his own. I know that same feeling of "wretchedness" all too well.

But here's the hope. Just a few verses later, Paul wrote, "Therefore, there is now no condemnation for those who are in Christ Jesus" (Romans 8:1–2 NIV). Paul had condemned himself, but Jesus hadn't. The difference between Paul and me is that Paul let the scarcity he felt push him deeper into the grace of God.

You *will* have moments of weakness and hopelessness. There will be things that you face in your life—whether it be addiction, an eating disorder, or a particular pattern of sin—that will make you feel insufficient. This is what it means to be human, living in a fallen world.

But the good news? It's Jesus. His abundance fills in the gaps of our scarcity.

Where we are bound to the scarcity mentality of "I will never be enough," the power of Jesus abounds all the more. God's Word assures us so.

His
abundance
fills in the
gaps of our
scarcity.

When Paul asked for healing, God lovingly replied, "'My grace is sufficient for you, for my power is made perfect in weakness.' Therefore I will boast all the more gladly of my weaknesses, so that Christ's power may rest on me" (2 Corinthians 12:8–9 NIV).

Whenever you feel like you can't get past your faults, when you feel reeled back into a temptation you'd sworn off, when you realize that your own strength is not enough, focus your eyes on the truth that God loves you beyond measure. Jesus calls you worthy of His pursuit, worthy of His love, and worthy of His resurrection power. He is chasing after you with eternal hope that can conquer any struggle you face. No amount of our "not enough-ness" can stop His love.

If you feel like I did that day with my arms wrapped around a toilet seat, believing that despair is more powerful than the Light, your downward spiral might feel swift and powerful. Be encouraged that it is precisely in that lowly state—in that gap of your insufficiency—that you have a front-row seat to God's sufficiency. This moment of weakness is what matters. Will you look up from that dark pit you're in and see the God who is trying to get you out? If you are headed there, just look up! Know that even in your moments of despair, the abundant power of Christ will burn all the brighter.

Lord,

To get out of the pit of hopelessness, I must first realize that I am in it. I set my eyes on my need for You and the truth that I am not enough in my own strength. Make Your abundant power known in the despair that I feel. When I am at my weakest, Your strength remains unchanged. Help me not get stuck here, God; help me see Your hand, reaching down to save and redeem.

Amen.

He Has
Rescued
Us.

The Gospel of Enough

Can you see Him? Reaching down to pull you out of the pit? I know it's dark. You didn't mean to fall—you got distracted, looking at the wrong thing, and next thing you knew, you were tumbling down into this abyss. It hadn't yet occurred to you to look up, back the way you came.

Look up. There's the Light.

Set your eyes higher. That's the world you belong to up there.

Reach out your hand; He's been waiting for you to hear to His voice, to turn around and grab on so He can lift you out.

He did it for me, and He will do the same for you, no matter what you're facing today. No pit of despair is too much for Jesus.

> I waited patiently for the LORD;
> he turned to me and heard my cry.
> He lifted me out of the slimy pit,
> out of the mud and mire;
> he set my feet on a rock

and gave me a firm place to stand.
He put a new song in my mouth,
a hymn of praise to our God.

Psalm 40:1–3 NIV

When we find ourselves in the pit of despair, as all of us will at some point in our lives, we must first allow ourselves to process the pain.

Then we let God lift us from it.

I remember my low moments, longing to feel like I was worthy and like I was enough. If I could perform perfectly at work or school and make everyone happy and earn others' admiration and feel attractive (physically, socially, and, of course, romantically), maybe *then* I would believe that I was worthy of God's love. Maybe then I would start to live like it.

Unfortunately, if you're waiting to *feel* sufficient, you will always be waiting. For me to finally feel like I was enough, I needed to look at the love of Jesus. The solution to my internal scarcity was to stop looking at myself and to start looking at the abundance found in *Him*.

So I want to share the gospel with you today: Jesus died on the cross to restore you to health and free you into abundant, joyful living. God has never *needed* you to be good enough; His Son bore the burden for you. Not only that, but God, in His rich mercy, decided in His own steadfast love that you were enough for that history-altering, earth-shattering sacrifice. God didn't choose Israel as His own because they were a perfect nation; He chose them because when this small, otherwise insignificant people flourished (often against all odds), it pointed to His power and steadfast love (Deuteronomy 7:7–9; 1 Corinthians 1:26–31). That's the design for your life too. As the gospel always is, this message is profoundly countercultural, but when you embrace the knowledge you need a Savior, you will experience fresh abundance and joy.

The nuance here matters so much: you are not enough *on your own*, and it's important to earnestly grapple with the theological reality of that. Even the very best of you—your wisdom, beauty, or power—will eventually fade, wither, and fail. Just like Israel, we are small and insignificant in the grand scheme of things, and no amount of our striving will change that. Yet in spite of that, Jesus died for you because *He* decided that you were enough. Now, you get to live from that enough-ness. God made you "enough" so now *you are.*

Your despair meets its end in Christ Jesus, Savior of the world.

I have never been strong enough to climb out of the pit by myself. In fact, most of the time, I find myself digging the pit deeper, shovel in hand. When it comes to that slimy pit from Psalm 40, I am unable to help myself—the definition of "not enough."

But Jesus has chosen to sit at the edge, calling my name. The Conqueror of death and the King of heaven has decided I am worth His time, that I am enough to Him. *"For he has rescued us from the dominion of darkness* and brought us into the kingdom of the Son he loves, in whom we have redemption, the forgiveness of sins" (Colossians 1:13–14 NIV, emphasis added). He has taken my place and traded my burden, and that's the kind of abundance He's calling you into right now. Set your eyes higher.

Lord,
I see You there, reaching down to lift me
from my despair. I am not enough. I am so scared
that I am not enough. But for that, I will praise
You all the more. You have decided to make me
worthy; You have decided that I am enough. I
am setting my eyes higher, squarely on Your
love and mercy for me. Thank You, Lord Jesus.
Amen.

Afterword

Since, then, you have been raised with Christ, set
your hearts on things above, where Christ is, seated
at the right hand of God. Set your minds on things
above, not on earthly things. For you died, and your
life is now hidden with Christ in God. When Christ,
who is your life, appears, then you also will appear
with him in glory.

Colossians 3:1–4 NIV

This is what setting our eyes higher has been about.

According to Colossians 3, Christ is on the throne, and our
hearts are set on that reality. And if we know and believe that
Christ is at the Father's right hand, our minds, too, are oriented
to this reality.

Our hearts and minds are set to heaven, so why do we struggle
to live that way?

We still inhabit physical bodies and limited minds, which
cause us to struggle to see past the reality in front of our eyes. We
must learn to set them higher too.

When you find yourself struggling to believe that your identity
is secure, you must intentionally set your eyes on God's image and
the profound value and intentionality He has woven into you too.

When your mind is rattling with information, making it all too easy to believe that you need to have all the answers—look up and focus instead on God's wisdom.

When you feel weighed down by the infinite burden of trying to fix the world in your own strength—and the intense, debilitating burnout that often follows—focus on His power and the small, beautiful missions He is inviting you into for the good of the world.

When it feels like there isn't enough money, time, or opportunities, set your eyes on His provision. When you feel like you aren't enough, set your eyes on His love.

For the past forty days, setting our eyes higher has been a daily practice. The world wants your eyes low; make an intentional practice of eternal perspective and humility before our great God. He wants your good, and the good of all creation. He wants your flourishing, so that He might use you for the flourishing of others. He is at work in mighty ways, if only our eyes are trained to see.

Go on from here, but don't stop looking up. Each and every day, set those beautiful eyes higher. I promise you'll see Him, and I promise it will change everything.

Bibliography

Champagne Butterfield, Rosaria. *The Gospel Comes with a House Key: Practicing Radically Ordinary Hospitality in Our Post-Christian World*. (Wheaton: Crossway, 2018).

Comer, John Mark. *The Ruthless Elimination of Hurry*. (Colorado Springs: Waterbrook, 2019).

Dennison, Kara. "Executives and Leaders Are Leaving Their Roles due to Burnout." *Forbes*. Published March 31, 2022. Accessed October 26, 2023. https://www.forbes.com/sites/karadennison/2022/07/28/executives-and-leaders-are-leaving-their-roles-due-to-burnout/?sh=4a8f17a6db95.

Fadling, Alan. *An Unhurried Life: Following Jesus' Rhythms of Work and Rest*. (Westmont: InterVarsity Press, 2020).

Foster, Richard J. "Book Excerpt: Understanding Solitude." Renovaré. Renovare.org. Updated July 2023. https://renovare.org/articles/understanding-solitude#:~:text=Silence%2C%20you%20see%2C%20creates%20in,%E2%80%8B"towers%20of%20babble."

Graham, Carol. "America's Crisis of Despair: A Federal Task Force for Economic Recovery and Societal Well-Being." Brookings. Published February 10, 2021. https://www.brookings.edu/articles

/americas-crisis-of-despair-a-federal-task-force-for-economic
-recovery-and-societal-well-being/.

"New CDC Data Illuminate Youth Mental Health Threats during
the COVID-19 Pandemic." Centers for Disease Control and
Prevention (CDC). Published March 31, 2022. https://www.cdc
.gov/media/releases/2022/p0331-youth-mental-health-covid-19
.html.

"New Surgeon General Advisory Raises Alarm about the Devastating
Impact of the Epidemic of Loneliness and Isolation in the United
States." US Department of Health and Human Services (HHS).
Published May 3, 2023. https://www.hhs.gov/about/news/2023/05
/03/new-surgeon-general-advisory-raises-alarm-about-devastating
-impact-epidemic-loneliness-isolation-united-states.html.

Oxford Languages, s.v. "cynicism," accessed February 9, 2024, https://
doi.org/10.1093/OED/1385922087.

Park, Ju-Hyeon, Young-Woo Seo, and Seungbum Chae. "Impact
of the COVID-19 Pandemic on Adolescent Self-Harm: Based
on a National Emergency Department Information System."
International Journal of Environmental Research and Public Health.
Ed. Paul B. Tchounwou. March 6, 2023. https://doi.org/10.3390
/ijerph20054666.

Segal, Marshall ed. *Killjoys: The Seven Deadly Sins.* (Minneapolis:
Desiring God, 2015).

Wheelwright, Trevor. "Cell Phone Behavior Survey: Are People
Addicted to Their Phones?" Reviews.org. January 24, 2022. https://
www.reviews.org/mobile/cell-phone-addiction/.

About the Author

Whitney Lowe is a Christian influencer who wants to see young women excited about God's work: in the Bible, in history, in the world, and in them. She writes and creates on Instagram @ScribbleDevos, a project born from the realization that young women simply do not interact with the Bible enough to be changed by its truth. Whitney is passionate about disrupting the toxic scroll of social media with hope, peace, and light straight from Scripture. She lives in Denver, Colorado, with her husband, who is a pastor, and their two young children.

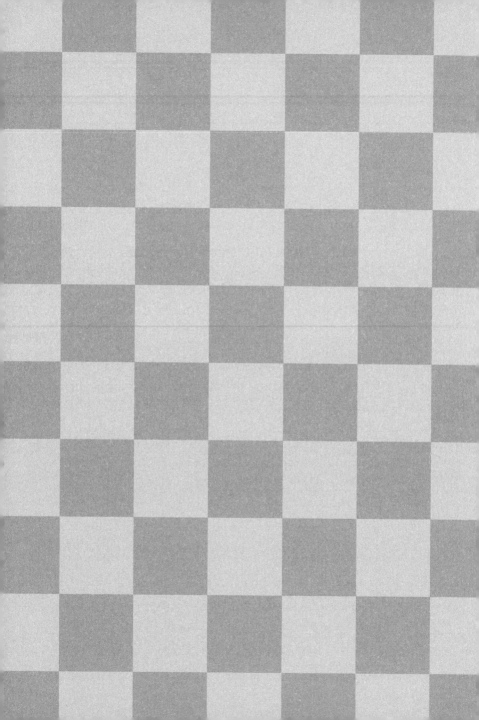